t'ai chi

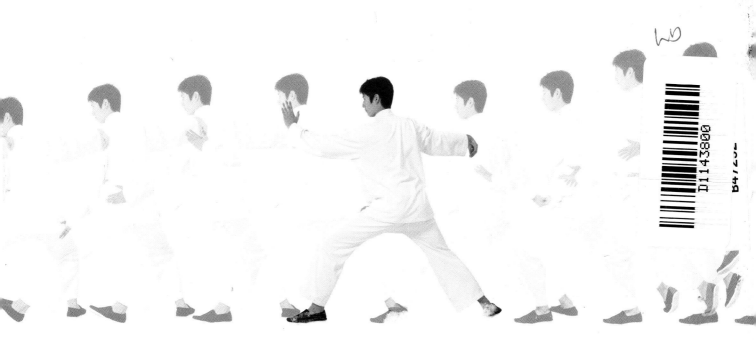

a *flowmotion* title

t'ai chi

yang style 24-move short form

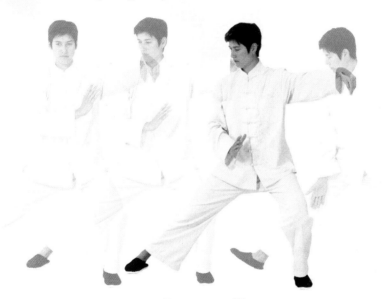

James Drewe

A CONNECTIONS • AXIS EDITION

A Connections • Axis Edition

First edition published in Great Britain by
Connections Book Publishing Limited
St Chad's House
148 King's Cross Road
London WC1X 9DH
and Axis Publishing Limited
8c Accommodation Road
London NW11 8ED
www.axispublishing.co.uk

First reprinted in 2002

Conceived and created by
Axis Publishing Limited

Creative Director: Siân Keogh
Managing Editor: Matthew Harvey
Project Designer: Juliet Brown
Project Editor: Madeleine Jennings
Photographer: Mike Good

Text and images copyright
© Axis Publishing Limited 2002

Note
The opinions and advice expressed in this book
are intended as a guide only. The publisher and
author accept no responsibility for any
injury or loss sustained as a result of
using this book.

British Library Cataloguing-in-Publication
data available on request.

ISBN 1–85906–081–1

9 8 7 6 5 4 3

Separation by United Graphics Pte Limited
Printed and bound by Star Standard (Pte) Limited

a *flow*motion title
t'ai chi

contents

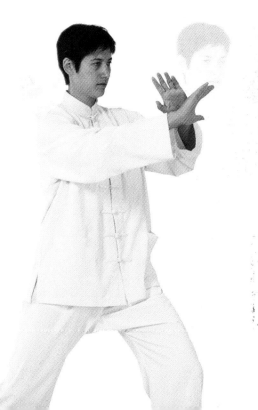

foreword

The purpose of this book is to provide a guide for anyone wishing to learn the shape of the t'ai chi 24-move Beijing short form. T'ai chi, taiji, t'ai chi ch'uan and taijiquan are all the same discipline. T'ai chi ch'uan translates as 'supreme ultimate fist', or 'the way of supreme harmony.' T'ai chi is the shortened version. The majority of people practising t'ai chi in the West do so mainly for health reasons, but there is also a self-defence application. A good t'ai chi class should also include the self-defence aspect because only through understanding the moves in their entirety will one be able to direct the flow of energy correctly through the body. It is not clear from what date the discipline originates, but it is thought to have been developed into something resembling its current form in the 18th and 19th centuries. There are many styles of t'ai chi, such as the Chen, Yang, Wu, Sun and Hao styles, and these names all refer to the families from which the style originates. The Yang style is arguably the most popular style at the moment, but the Chen style is becoming a close second.

why do t'ai chi?

T'ai chi is commonly practised for its health benefits. The Chinese believe that the vital energy in all life (known as ch'i or qi) flows through each of us, and that the amount of ch'i we each have determines our health. This ties in with the theory of acupuncture in which the body's energy moves in a series of channels or meridians, and that the health of the individual is determined by the condition of the channels and related organs. If a person suffers from stress, which blocks the flow of ch'i, they may become tired more easily and be more susceptible to physical problems such as bowel disorders, headaches, poor circulation, fatigue or high blood pressure. T'ai chi aims to allow the body to open up, the muscles to relax, the tissues to expand and the joints to open and connect, so that the ch'i can flow more freely through the body. Once this starts to happen, you feel greatly energised and it becomes increasingly easier to relax.

However, there is a further benefit. As the body starts to relax and the energy can be felt moving through the body, the energy is not used up but actually starts to accumulate in the Dantian – an area of the body centred approximately two inches below the navel and about a third of the way into the body. The Dantian acts as a storehouse of ch'i. This generation and collection of energy is why t'ai chi is known as an exercise for increasing energy and building stamina.

will I damage myself doing t'ai chi?

As long as you don't try to push yourself by competing with others when doing t'ai chi, you stand little chance of hurting yourself. The most common injury when doing t'ai chi is damage to the knees, and this is why a competent teacher is important from the beginning, before you have formed bad habits. If you are attempting t'ai chi without a teacher, to be safe, never allow the knee to go beyond the toes, and always keep the knee in the centre of the line of pressure from the pelvis to the foot (that is, don't allow the knee to collapse inwards or outwards).

practising alone and with others

It is important to find a teacher when you learn t'ai chi, as the art involves much more than just a series of movements. The majority of people are unaware of their posture and balance, and many do not know how to relax, so a trained, experienced teacher is essential for the beginner. However, if you are learning at home in order to get the feel of the movements, there is no initial harm in practising without expert guidance – just copy the postures as accurately as possible.

There is no specified amount of time to practise – it should be as often as possible, but never so that you become tired. It is advantageous to practise with other people, who can help with motivation and with moves that you cannot remember; however, the disadvantages are that others may want to go much faster than you, or may be doing the moves entirely wrong. We recommend that you combine approaches, both working with others and alone. Practising alone is absolutely essential, because it is only

then that you will find out whether or not you really understand the moves. Many people worry that they might practise the moves incorrectly. There is more value in practising a move incorrectly, than in not practising at all; it is only through trial and error that you will learn to practise the moves correctly. Throughout your practice it is important to stay open to the possibility that it might not be right – this will make it that much easier to adjust to the correction.

the benefits of t'ai chi

Learning the form will teach you the best possible way in which to align your body so that your energy will flow unimpeded. This has several beneficial effects: you will feel better both physically and mentally, you will feel more relaxed, you will be better coordinated, you will have found a way to release stress and tension, you will feel more grounded and better connected to the world around you, you will feel warmer, certain physical problems may disappear, your muscles will become toned with regular practise, your posture and balance will improve, you may not become ill so often because an increased flow of energy will strengthen you, you will be calmer but more alert, you may become better at decision making and you might find that you gain in confidence.

After a t'ai chi class you should feel well exercised, but, unlike other forms of exercise, which may leave you feeling tired and needing to rest, you will feel refreshed, revitalised and relaxed. This is because t'ai chi incorporates exercises that help to control and develop your ch'i rather than just develop your muscles.

energy within the body

CH'I OR QI The flow of vital energy is often first experienced in the palms and fingers as a sensation of warmth. This may be accompanied by a tingling sensation, and/or a feeling of swelling as though the hands have become bigger. As you increasingly relax, this feeling can extend to the feet and eventually to the entire body.

THE MIND While doing t'ai chi, the mind should be relaxed and calm. This can be extremely difficult for people who are beginners, as they are constantly having to assess their movements and coordinate their weight, legs, arms, hands, toes, body turn and eyes. At the same time, they have to check that not only is the basic posture correct, but that the stance which they are attempting to achieve is also correct. This explains why it is important to repeat each move over and over again, so that the body's own intelligence (as opposed to the mind's) can learn the moves, and the moves become instinctive.

BREATHING As you learn the t'ai chi form, the correct breathing will develop automatically. It is initially better not to assign a breath (inhalation or exhalation) to a particular move of the form, as this can encourage the breath to become forced. Once you become familiar with the form however, it will become apparent straightaway which moves require an inhalation or exhalation. Generally, although there are a few exceptions, you inhale on the yin (contracting) movements, and exhale on the yang (expanding) movements. However, focus on the movements first – yin and yang awareness will come with greater experience.

EYES The eyes are one way of leading the energy through the body. Many movements require the eyes to turn in a certain direction, or to look at a particular hand during a movement. The Chinese extend this further to refer to the Yi or the 'intention' of a move, which makes the ch'i connect to a particular part of the body. This is easily felt in any pushing movement, during which you should feel that you are actually pushing something (but with relaxed muscles), even though there is nothing there to push.

SELF-DEFENCE It is worth looking at the self-defence applications of the moves, if only because they make the intention of the moves clearer. This will help your energy travel around the body in a more controlled manner, and in a way of which you can become more easily aware.

using the waist – working from the centre

The waist controls every move that the hands make, and the feet control every move that the waist makes. In t'ai chi it is said, 'Energy is initiated in the feet, controlled and directed by the waist and manifested in the hands'. Any hand movement must come from this central point. For example, if the arms go out to the right side, the waist must turn to the right a split second beforehand. 'The waist' really refers to the Dantian: This should be like a sphere inside you that rotates and causes the arms to move. The body continuously revolves as your weight shifts forwards and backwards.

opening and closing

The arms and legs also have a system of 'breathing'. When one elbow moves away from the other you are opening on that side, but when it comes towards the other, you are closing on that side. In the legs, the opening or closing is governed by the Kua, or the 'inguinal groove' in the pelvis. This is the crease to the left and right of the pelvis where the thighs meet the pelvis. If you stand with your feet together and then rotate one knee out sideways without turning your body, you are opening the Kua.

On a more advanced level, the opening and closing is governed by what is known as the 'bows' of the arms and legs (see below). This is a feeling of connection between, for example, the hands on both sides, from the fingertips of one hand, up the arm, across the shoulders and down the other arm to the fingertips of the other hand. It is called a 'bow' precisely because it resembles a bow. When the hands move towards each other, there should be a feeling of the ends of the wooden bow being bent. In other words, there should be the same sensation of latent power within the finger-shoulders-finger structure as there is in a bow that is being compressed ready to release an arrow.

In a closing action, with the palms moving towards each other, this feeling of connection or latent power should be maintained, so that if both your arms are now out in front of you, and someone were to push one of your hands towards you, you should also feel the push in the other hand as the energy travels around the back. The same feeling can be achieved in the legs by linking them through the arch of the pelvis.

connections

There are three important directions of connection within the body:

1. Top to bottom

2. Left to right

3. Front to back: this means that as you push your wrist away, there is a simultaneous expansion backwards with the upper part of the back. This backward expansion may or may not be visible, but should be there all the same, connecting your wrist to your back.

ON THE INSIDE
While it might look simple from the outside, getting the inner aspects of t'ai chi right can take years of practise. The benefits more than make up for the effort.

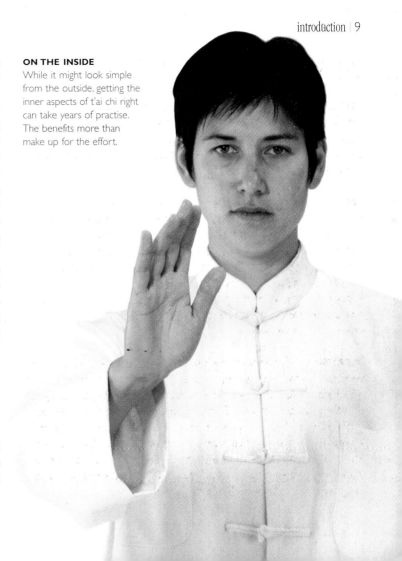

T'AI CHI HANDS

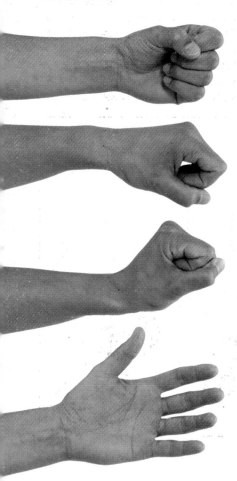

T'AI CHI FIST
When a fist is used in t'ai chi, the hand is not clenched. You should feel energy focused at the hand and flowing freely.

GOOD FIST
There is a finger-sized hole within the fingers – the 'eye' of the fist. The knuckles and forearm are aligned.

BAD FIST
Clenching the fist too tightly causes an energy blockage and can affect the rest of your posture and movement.

T'AI CHI HAND
When not in a specified position, the hand should be neither rigid nor floppy, allowing energy to flow freely. Usually, the fingers are spread slightly apart, with the palm open as though resting on a beach ball.

relaxation, softness, and the muscles

T'ai chi movement should be completely soft and totally relaxed. Tensed muscles contract, shrinking the muscles and hardening the body. To relax in t'ai chi means that one allows the muscles to 'lengthen' – there is an expansion with direction. In many moves you also allow the limbs and/or body to widen, as though, for example, the arms are getting wider as well. Many beginners have difficulty relaxing their shoulders. Once the shoulders are relaxed a profound change comes over the entire body in that the body connects better. It is often quite helpful to think of relaxing the shoulder blades, rather than the shoulders. Therefore when doing any kind of pushing move, as you push, feel the muscles of the arms lengthening as you allow the shoulder blades to sink and widen.

This way of moving the muscles means that a different element of the muscle comes into play. Muscle fibres come in two kinds: fast twitching and slow twitching. The first are generally more powerful and are used when doing high-performance, short-duration exercise. Slow-twitching muscles are for endurance and are better for low-performance, long-duration exercises. In t'ai chi, the body comes to rely more on the slow-twitch fibres to sustain power and movement.

yin and yang in the form

All moves in the form have a yin or yang quality and contain aspects of both. However, all moves have one dominant characteristic, the yin moves being those that contract, sink or move inwards, and the yang moves being those that expand, rise or move outwards. Yang will always turn into yin, and vice versa – this is how the form 'breathes'. To visualise this movement, you need to see every event in the form as initiating from the 'centre', i.e. the Dantian. Therefore, not only do the movements themselves flow inwards and outwards from the centre, but the individual parts of the body, which make up the moves, also 'breathe' within their own separate sequence of movements. The whole form consists of a series of inward and outward, or yin and yang, movements.

For example, the arms not only extend forwards and backwards but also open and close sideways. They also have the ability to rotate (spiral) as they move inwards and outwards. The legs do the same: the weight not only shifts forwards and backwards, but the knees spiral outwards on certain moves, and the Kua opens and closes, usually opening on one side while closing on the other. The back, across the shoulder blades, continuously opens and closes with every outward and inward movement – another aspect of the yin and yang of the form. When all of the yin and yang changes occur simultaneously, there is a feeling of the entire body 'breathing', in addition to the breathing of the lungs themselves.

SLIPPING THE HEEL

This is the movement of the rear foot used to get into the bow stance. During this move, most of the weight is on the other foot. This allows you to realign the foot without taking it off the floor.
To perform the slip heel, ensure that about 70 per cent of your weight is on the front foot. Throughout the movement, you will keep the rear foot completely flat.
Imagine that the part of your foot just behind the toes (the ball) is the pivot of the movement, fixed to the floor. As your body moves, rotate on this pivot, sliding the heel around. The toes will also move in the opposite direction, but the ball of the foot should remain over the same spot. As you perform the heel slip, your knee will also move – keep this flexed and loose, but keep some weight on it.

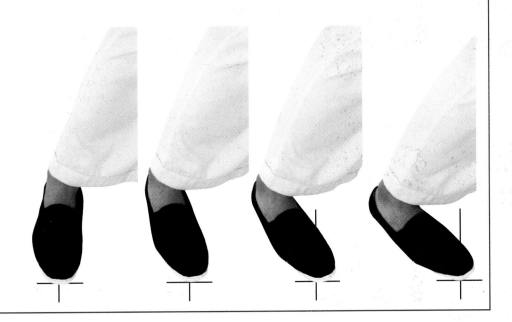

the basic upright posture

The ability to relax stems from correct posture. For example, if your upper body is constantly leaning or slumped forwards, it is impossible to relax the muscles in the back and at the back of the pelvis. You need to achieve a posture that requires the minimum effort to keep you upright; this could be compared to dishes being stacked high on the draining board – they need to be vertical to stop them from falling over.

1. Stand with your feet shoulder-width apart, your body upright with the weight evenly distributed between both feet and towards the centre of each foot.

2. Relax your feet, particularly in the instep of the foot, and as you do so, allow the toes to lengthen ahead of you. Rest the toes on the floor.

3. Consciously relax every joint in the body from the ankles upwards; the knees should be straight – this means that they should neither be bent forwards, nor locked backwards.

4. Soften the pelvis to rest on the thighs and relax the waist and abdomen. The shoulder blades should feel as though they are connected to the feet (try feeling the weight of the

shoulders falling into the feet). Allow the shoulders to widen so that the muscles across the chest and back are released.

5. The fingers and palms should hang on either side of you with the weight of the hands only stretching the arms downwards. This will allow the shoulder, elbow and wrist joints to release and open.

6. The body also needs to make a vertical expansion. Now allow the neck to release and relax from the seventh cervical vertebra (the most prominent bone just above the level of the shoulders) up to the Atlas joint that meets the skull high up at the back of the head. The action of relaxing the neck will cause the crown of the head to rise.

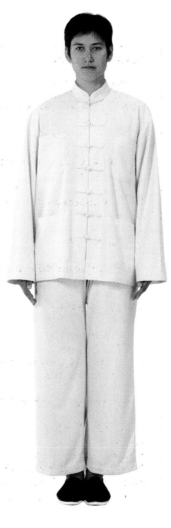

THE BASIC T'AI CHI POSTURE INVOLVES THE FOLLOWING:

- Relax the neck to raise the crown of the head.

- Relax the chest and straighten the back.

- Relax the waist and small of the back, allowing the tailbone to tuck under.

- Relax the hips and pelvis.

- Release the shoulders (shoulder blades) and elbows.

- Drop the fingers by your sides, allowing them to lengthen from the elbow.

- Keep the spine upright, but without any tension.

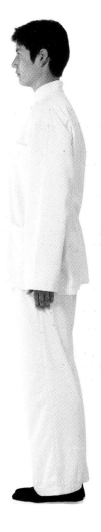

FAULTS IN POSTURE

1. Neck bent forward.

2. Highest point of the head leaning in any direction.

3. Raised shoulders, unrelaxed shoulder blades.

4. Elbows raised in such a way as to cause the shoulders to rise.

5. Back hunched, causing the spine to collapse and disconnect.

6. Collapsed chest.

7. Pelvis tilting so that the small of the back disconnects (unstable waist).

8. Buttocks protruding.

9. Hips unaligned.

10. Pelvis protruding forwards, often caused by the body leaning backwards.

11. Locked knees (hyper-extended).

12. The sole of the foot is not in complete contact with the floor. This is not the same as the heel being raised as in some moves (for example, White Crane Spreads its Wings) or the toe being raised as in other moves (for example, Play the Lute).

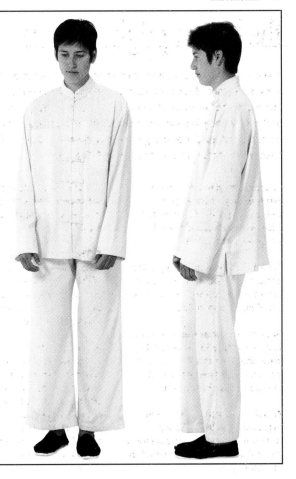

key stances and posture

the bow of the arms

The body must be centred; therefore in flexion the flexibility of the arms is equal on both sides. The shoulders should sink so that both shoulders and arms connect centrally to the spine.

The elbows should sink so the connection to the wrists is completed, which also allows the shoulders to relax. Generally, the elbows stay lower than the shoulders. The elbow joints should never be less than 90 degrees. However, there are some exceptions to this; for example, the 'folding' arm in Brush Knee and Side Step, or the 'folding' arm in Repulse Monkey.

The wrists should be straight but relaxed so that the connection to the fingertips is completed. When the upper arms are down, there should always be a space under the armpits. The arms are always held in a gentle curve. The palms are slightly concave, as though holding a large beach ball.

the bow of the legs

The buttocks and tailbone should be tucked in. This allows the spine to straighten, the neck to lengthen, and allows the pelvis and upper body to connect to the legs. There should be no tension in the abdomen. The bow of the leg is most apparent when the body is in the Bow Stance (see p. 15).

stances

All stances come from the basic posture, and all the principles of the above should be put into practise when moving from one stance to another. The main difference between the basic posture and the stance is that in the latter there is a transfer of weight from one bent leg to the other.

Whatever style of t'ai chi one is learning, it is important to be clear about the distribution of weight in the stance. It is as though one leg is full of water and the other leg is empty – when you move from one position to another, the water pours from one leg to the other. Usually 60–70 per cent of the weight is on one leg.

T-STEP STANCE

The weight is entirely on one foot. The other foot is drawn close to the ankle of the supporting foot with the toe pointing downwards. The toe does not necessarily have to be suspended in the air – it can lightly rest on the floor by the side of the supporting foot.

This is always an intermediate move. The 'empty' foot is generally either in the process of stepping or rising up for a kick.

NOTE: Beginners make the error of placing weight on the toes of the foot that is touching the floor.

BOW STANCE

The front leg is bent with 60–70 per cent of the weight resting on it. The back leg is very slightly bent like a bow before it is drawn. The back foot should be 45 degrees to the front foot. The sole of the back foot is firmly planted on the floor.

The stance should have the feet well separated to the left and right – this is rather as though you are walking on railway lines with a foot on each rail – but with one foot ahead of the other.

NOTE: When using the bow stance, most beginners make the stance too narrow, and lift the little toe of the rear foot.

Examples of this stance can be seen in Parting the Wild Horse's Mane, Brush Knee and Side Step, and Peng (in Grasp the Sparrow's Tail).

EMPTY STANCES

The T-Step stance could be called an empty stance, as it is 'empty' in one leg. However, conventionally, the empty stances have one leg extended ahead with either the sole of the foot flat, or with the heel or toes touching the floor. In the empty stances, the standing leg is bent. The knee of the extended leg is also slightly bent.

NOTE: Most beginners make the error of leaning the body backwards in this stance.

Examples of this stance can be seen in Stork Spreads its Wings, Play The Lute and Repulse Monkey.

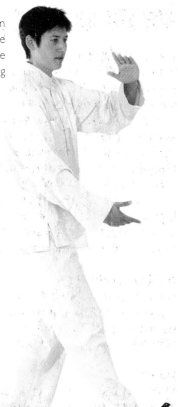

peng jing

This can be loosely translated as 'ward-off energy'. Peng Jing could be compared to your body being surrounded by a very large rubber ball – when someone pushes you, it will feel to them as though they are pushing something resilient, something that gives slightly but is still firm. It is a quality of strength and flexibility. With correct posture and stance, the body becomes surprisingly powerful; for example, when being pushed, it can feel as though there is no one pushing at all, regardless of the force being applied. To a certain extent this is true, because if there is a very good connection of the body, and the alignment is correct, in effect the energy of the push passes through you, and you almost cease to become involved. It feels as though the energy of the person pushing is just passing into and through your back foot and pushing the earth beneath your foot.

MOVING FROM A LEFT BOW STANCE TO A RIGHT BOW STANCE

This movement takes place in sequences such as Parting the Wild Horse's Mane and Brush Knee and Side Step.

Face nine o'clock, left foot forward. Sit back on your right foot, turn your body to face 7.30, raising the left toes and turning them towards 7.30. Move your body forwards over your left foot (which is still facing 7.30).

Bring your right foot into your left foot (T-Step intermediate foot move). Place your right foot ahead of you with toes pointing towards nine o'clock, but remember to widen your stance as though walking on railway lines; there is no weight on the right foot as yet (this is an empty stance).

Move your weight forwards onto your right foot. Your back foot will automatically be correctly angled at 45 degrees to the front foot because you turned it to 7.30 previously.

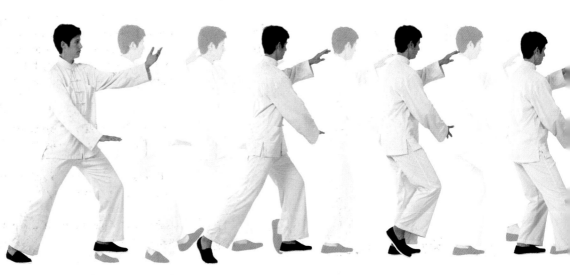

Performing t'ai chi ch'uan movements:

Remember that all movements should be

performed with relaxation and sinking;

performed with gentleness and softness, yet with intention,

continuous, flowing and even circular or curving motions.

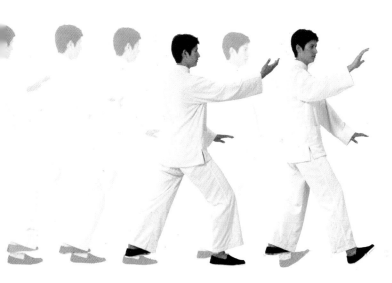

WHEN PRACTISING

1. Keep your attention focused on every movement, as this will enhance the results of the exercise.

2. All the movements should be circular, relaxed and very soft. They should be performed slowly and smoothly. One movement should flow into the next in a continuous flow without apparent pauses – like 'silk being drawn from a cocoon'. In other words, the cocoon is your 'centre' – too hard a pull on the silk will break the thread.

3. Coordinate the movements of the head, body, arms, hands, legs, feet and eyes. Your body leads the movements of your limbs, while your waist acts as the hinge or main axis. The movements originate in the Dantian. If your body has to rise or lower it should do so gently. The movement of the whole body is interrelated.

4. Remember to breathe – it is easy to forget when concentrating intensely. Each breath should be deep and long, and should happen naturally with your movements.

5. Practise enough so as to feel exercised but not tired. This may be once or several times a day.

6. Practise slowly and make the movements even. The whole set takes 4–6 minutes.

names of the forms

The forms of the Yang-style 24-move short form make up a complete flowing sequence. When you have mastered the basic movements, you should try to perform the entire form in one session, without pauses.

When performed properly, the sequence should last about six minutes. The final direction of each form is listed next to the name of the form below. This system uses the clock face as a directional guide.

direction	form
12.00	1. Starting Form
9.00	2. Parting the Wild Horse's Mane on both sides
9.00	3. White Stork Spreads its Wings
9.00	4. Brush Knee and Side Step on both sides
9.00	5. Play the Lute (Guitar; Pippa)
3.00	6. Repulse Monkey
9.00	7. Grasp the Sparrow's Tail – left side
3.00	8. Grasp the Sparrow's Tail – right side
9.00	9. Single Whip
12.00	10. Wave Hands Like Clouds
9.00	11. Single Whip
9.00	12. High Pat on Horse

direction	form
10.00/10.30	13. Kick with Right Heel
10.30	14. Strike (Opponent's) Ears with Fists
4.30/5.00	15. Turn and Kick with Left Heel
3.00	16. Snake Creeps Down – Golden Cockerel – left
3.00	17. Snake Creeps Down – Golden Cockerel – right
4.30 & 1.30	18. Fair Lady Weaves her Shuttle on both sides
3.00	19. Needle at the Bottom of the Sea
3.00	20. Fan Through Back (Flash Arms)
9.00	21. Turn to Deflect Downwards, Parry and Punch
9.00	22. Apparent Close Up
12.00	23. Cross Hands
12.00	24. Closing (Finishing) Form

go with the flow

The special *Flowmotion* images used in this book have been created to ensure that you see the whole of each form – not just selected highlights. Each of the image sequences flows across the page from left to right, demonstrating how the form progresses and how to get into each position safely, effectively and with the appropriate flowing movement. The captions along the bottom of the images provide additional information to help you perform the forms confidently. Below this, another layer of information is contained in the timeline, including instructions for direction. As mentioned above, your breathing rhythm should fall naturally within the forms, inhaling on the yin stages and exhaling on the yang stages.

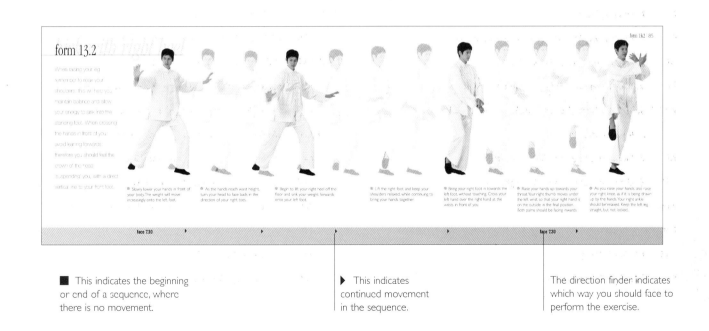

form 13.2

form 13.2 | 85

When raising your leg, remember not to raise your shoulders; this will help you maintain balance and allow your energy to sink into the standing foot. When crossing the hands in front of you, avoid leaning forwards; therefore you should feel the crown of the head suspending you, with a direct vertical line to your front foot.

■ Slowly lower your hands in front of your body. The weight will move increasingly onto the left foot.

■ As the hands reach waist height, turn your head to face back in the direction of your right toes.

■ Begin to lift your right heel off the floor and sink your weight forwards onto your left foot.

■ Lift the right foot and keep your shoulders relaxed, while continuing to bring your hands together.

■ Bring your right foot in towards the left foot, without touching. Cross your left hand over the right hand at the wrists in front of you.

■ Raise your hands up towards your throat. Your right thumb moves under the left wrist so that your right hand is on the outside in the final position. Both palms should be facing inwards

■ As you raise your hands and raise your right knee, as if it is being drawn up by the hands. Your right ankle should be relaxed. Keep the left leg straight, but not locked.

face 7.30   ▶   ▶   ▶   ▶   face 7.30   ▶

■ This indicates the beginning or end of a sequence, where there is no movement.

▶ This indicates continued movement in the sequence.

The direction finder indicates which way you should face to perform the exercise.

preparation for t'ai chi

preparatory exercise 1

The t'ai chi walk is one of the most fundamental techniques as it provides the link between many of the forms. It is important to be aware of both your balance and transfer of weight, and to ensure that, when stepping, you widen your stance as though walking on railway lines the width of your shoulders.

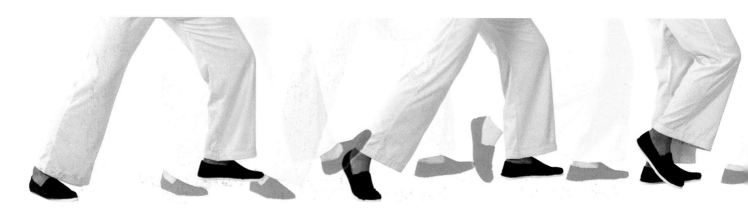

● Begin the movement in the left Bow Stance with your left foot forwards and bent at the knee, facing towards nine o'clock.

● Sit back onto your right foot and lift your left toes, turning them outwards, while at the same time turning your body to face 7.30. Transfer your weight onto the left foot.

● Now draw the right foot into the left foot (this is called the T-Step intermediate foot move).

● Now step ahead with the right foot, but widen your stance as though you are walking on railway lines, with your feet shoulder width apart.

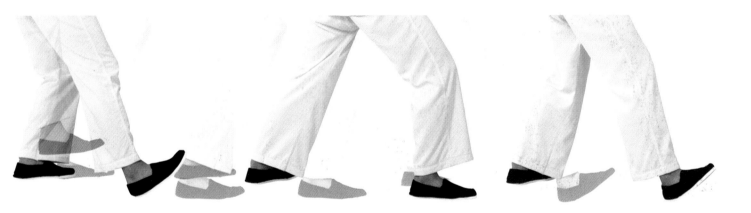

⬤ Transfer your weight forwards onto your right foot, lifting the toes up as you do so.

⬤ Place your foot down flat. The right toes should be pointing to nine o'clock, while the left foot is at a 45 degree angle to the right foot. This is called the right Bow Stance.

⬤ Now sit back with your weight onto the left foot and turn the toes of the right foot outwards.

⬤ Continue the t'ai chi walk, practicing both left and right Bow Stances consecutively.

preparatory exercise 2

The most important focus here is keeping the back straight as you shift your weight from one leg to the other. Keep your rear knee over the toes of your back foot and do not let it point inwards, which often happens when first practising the t'ai chi walk back.

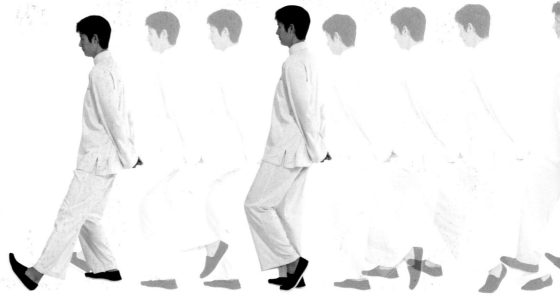

● Start by sitting back on your bent right leg with your right foot at a 45 degree angle. Your left leg should be stretched out in front, with the toes pointing up.

● Pick up the left foot and step back, resting it by the arch of the right foot. Keep your back straight. Next, step your left foot back, placing the toes in line with the right heel.

● Swivel on the ball of your left foot so that when you put the heel down, your foot is out at a 45 degree angle. Keep your left knee bent as you transfer the weight to the left leg and raise the toes of your right foot.

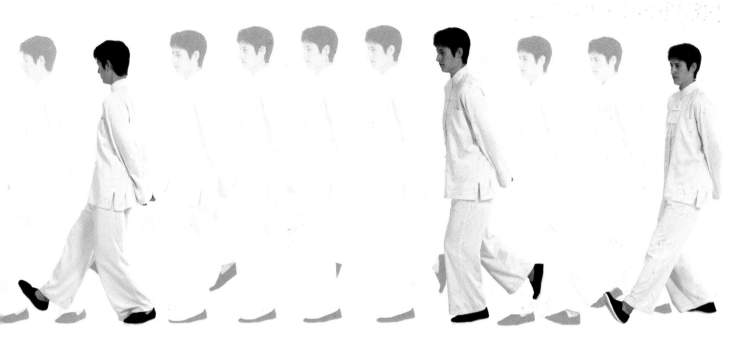

● Slowly pick up your right leg, and as you do so, turn your body so you are facing the 45 degree direction of your left foot. Try to maintain a straight back all the while.

● As for the previous side, gently rest the ball of your right foot by the middle of the left heel before taking it a step backwards.

● Swivel on the ball of your right heel so that when you place your right heel down on the floor, your foot is at a 45 degree angle.

● Lift the toes of your left foot towards the sky as you transfer the weight and sit back into the right leg.

warm up exercise 1

This warm up exercise will relax the knees, ankles, shoulders and wrists. The movement should be performed at a medium speed, and only take a few seconds. Repeat the movement at least 20 times for an effective warm up. Allow the Dantian to 'shake' slightly as you bounce.

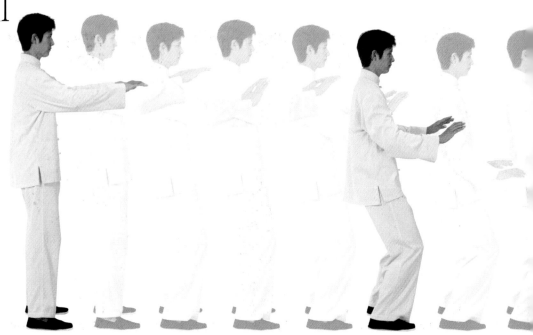

● To start the exercise, stand with your feet shoulder width apart and with your toes pointing forwards. Make sure your back is straight.

● Keep your shoulders and elbows relaxed and open. Slowly raise your arms up in front of you until they reach shoulder height.

● Drop your arms as you bend your knees, keeping your palms facing down towards the floor.

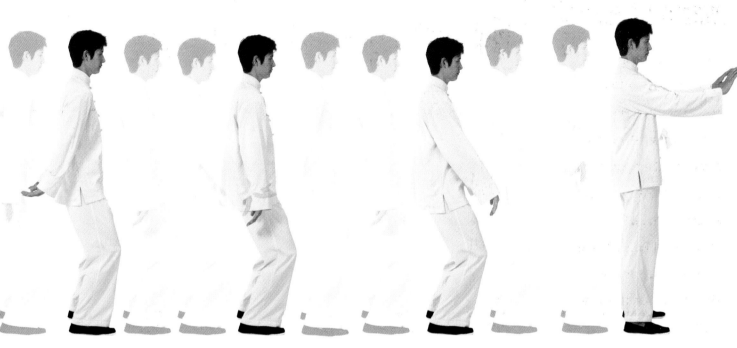

● Stand up about half way as you allow your hands to rise behind you. Keep your back straight.

● Bend your knees again and allow your arms to swing forwards, leading with your wrists soft at the joint.

● Start to raise your arms up in front of you again. Keep your shoulders down and your spine upright.

● Bring your arms up to shoulder height as you straighten your legs. Repeat this movement at least 20–100 times – each cycle should take just a few seconds.

▶ 12 o'clock   ▶   ▶ 12 o'clock   ■

warm up exercise 2.1

This exercise relaxes the shoulders, spine, knees and ankles, but above all the kua. As you sink and turn to the left, allow the kua to open on the right side and simultaneously close on the left side. This exercise, like the previous one, is not performed slowly; try to get some rhythm into the movement. For an effective warm up; repeat the exercise 20–100 times.

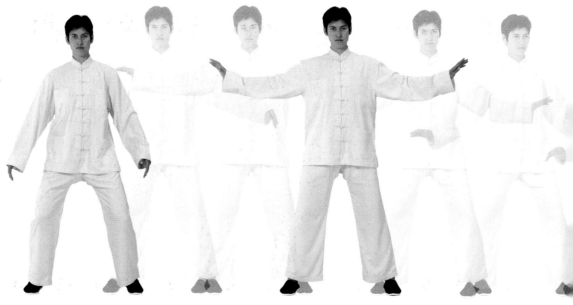

● Stand with your feet apart one and a half times your shoulder width. Hold your arms out to your sides, making sure they don't touch your body.

● Now raise your arms up on either side of your body to shoulder height. Keep your shoulders relaxed. You are now ready to start the exercise.

● Slowly bend your knees. Keep your back straight as you sink your weight down evenly between your legs. Slowly lower your arms.

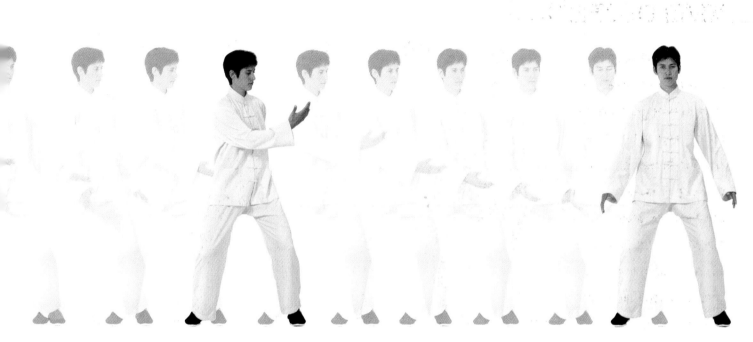

● Make sure your spine is upright as you begin to turn your body. Imagine a point of suspension on the crown of the head which is secured by a thread reaching up to the sky. This will help you to keep vertical as you move.

● Turn your head and body to the left as you bend your elbows and turn your palms to face the sky. Your right arm should swing in front of your body and the left one behind.

● Once you have turned as far as is comfortable, gradually lower your arm as you turn your head and body back to the front.

● Check your posture: your knees should be slightly bent so that you can maintain a low centre of gravity. Now repeat the movement 20–100 times.

warm up exercise 2.2

This exercise should only take a few seconds. It is important to remember that when you turn the body to the left or right, that you don't allow the back knee to collapse inwards. Keeping the knees open will avoid this problem. Keep the body vertical and, importantly, make sure that your weight doesn't move from foot to foot.

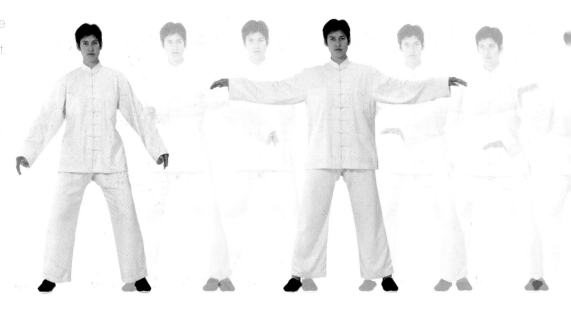

● Raise both arms up outwards to shoulder height. Your wrists should be soft at the joint.

● Keep your shoulders relaxed, making sure they don't rise in tandem with your arms. Raise your arms right up to shoulder height.

● Bend your knees as you start to sink downwards, lowering your arms as you do so and keeping your weight in the middle.

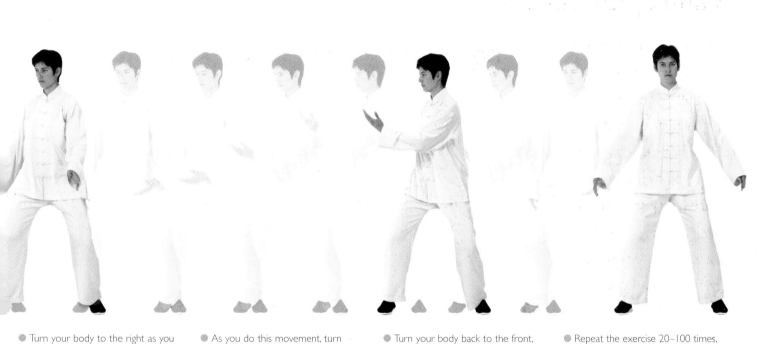

● Turn your body to the right as you bend your elbows and let your left arm swing in front of your body and your right arm swing behind.

● As you do this movement, turn your head to follow your left arm.

● Turn your body back to the front, lowering your arms to your side as you resume the start position.

● Repeat the exercise 20–100 times, remembering that the movement is performed at a medium speed.

warm up exercise 3

In this exercise, you should focus on keeping the body upright. The exercise involves vertically rotating the axis of the spine. Therefore, always keep the crown of the head above the midpoint between your feet. Ensure that it is the turn of the body that causes the arms to swing – the arms do not swing on their own.

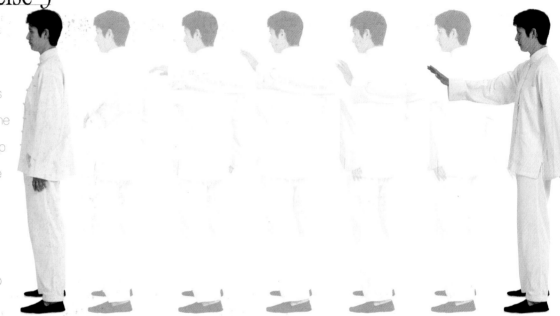

● Stand with your feet shoulder-width apart, back straight, shoulders relaxed and your gaze focused directly in front of you.

● Slowly turn your upper body to the right, but do not turn either your feet or head. As you turn, raise your left arm straight out in front of you to shoulder height.

● As your body turns, allow your right arm to swing behind you in a slow and controlled movement.

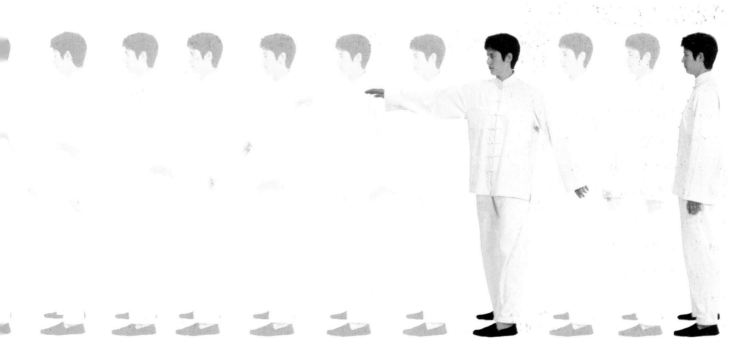

● Turn your body back around to the front. Swing the arms like a marching soldier, but using the turn of the body to create the swinging movement.

● Turn your body to your left, dropping your left arm and using the momentum of the swing to raise your right arm.

● Allow your left arm to swing slightly behind you as you raise your right arm to shoulder height. Keep your head still, but let your shoulders turn freely around either side.

● Repeat the sequence 20–100 times on both sides before returning to the centre with both arms by your sides.

▶   ▶   **turn to 10.30**   ▶   **face 12 o'clock** ■

form 1

starting form

This sequence consists of a preparatory movement followed by Form 1. The preparation elongates the body. You should be able to feel a vertical line running from the crown of your head down to your right foot. Remember to be very conscious of the shift in weight as you place the left foot under complete control.

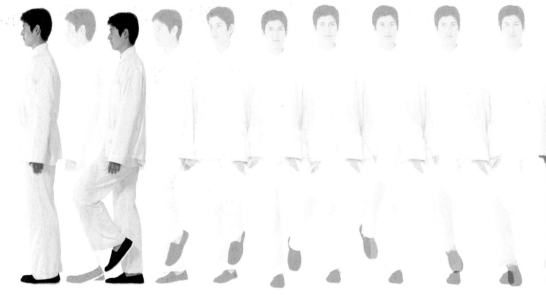

● To do the preparation, start with your feet together and your hands resting loosely by your side. Your back should be straight and your focus straight ahead with the crown of your head rising.

● Keep your focus and your arms to your side as you slowly raise your left heel and then the whole left leg.

● Step out with your left foot to shoulder width. Place the toes down first, followed by the heel. As your body weight transfers to the centre, your shoulders should be relaxed, square and balanced.

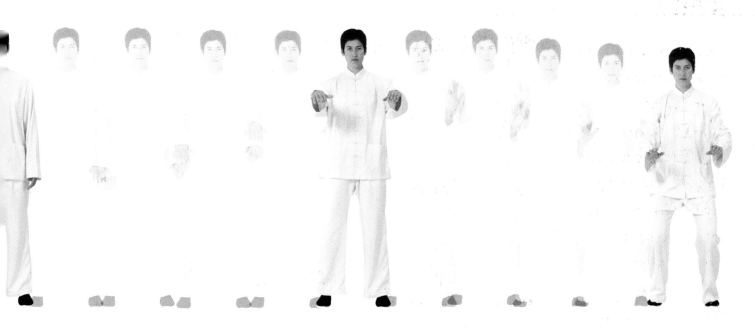

● Now begin Form 1. Slowly raise your wrists upwards and away in front of you, making sure that your fingers and palms are comfortably relaxed.

● Your wrists should now be at shoulder height. Check that your shoulders are relaxed and not hunched up round your ears.

● Simultaneously lower your forearms as you bend your knees. Keep your body in an upright position as you slowly sink down.

● The wrists should gently flex so that the fingers point slightly upwards as you sit. Lower the forearms until they are parallel to the ground, bringing the elbows back towards the body.

form 2.1

This form is repeated three times over the following pages: twice with the left hand extended, and once with the right hand extended. When you move your weight forwards into the final posture, you should feel that the extended hand is being pushed from the back foot.

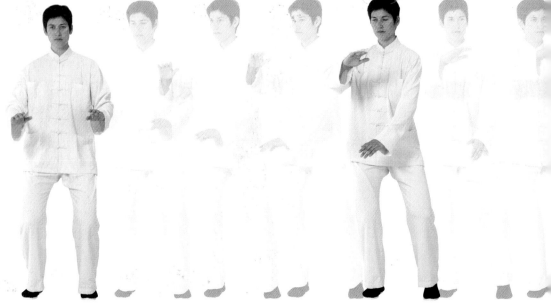

● Your body weight should be evenly distributed over both legs. Your back should be straight, your knees should be over your toes and your hands should be in line with your toes.

● Transfer your weight to your right foot and begin to turn in the direction of one o'clock.

● Raise the right hand up to shoulder height and move the left hand so that it is under the right hand. Start to turn the left palm upwards.

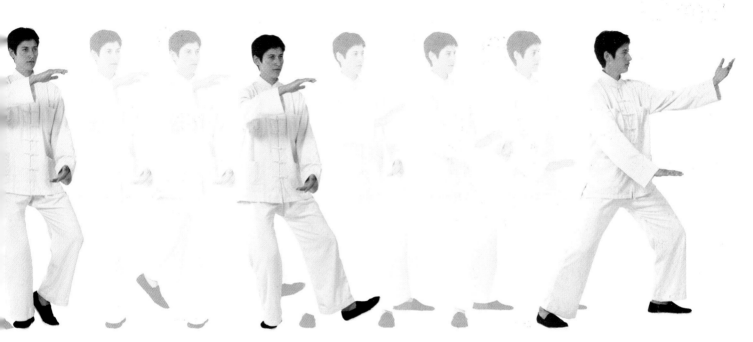

● Lift your left heel as you turn towards 10.30 and draw your left foot in to a T step as you finish turning your left hand as though holding a large imaginary ball. All three movements should be completed simultaneously.

● With all your weight on your right foot, step the left heel towards nine o'clock and widen your stance as though walking on railway lines that head towards nine o'clock.

● Transfer your weight on to your left foot, shift your weight forwards so that your left knee is bent over your left toes. Slip the right heel so that your right foot is at 45 degrees to your left foot with the left toes pointing towards nine o'clock.

● At the same time, move your right hand down so that the fingers are in line with the front of the right knee, and pointing towards nine o'clock. Raise your left hand so that the palm is facing diagonally upwards, with the arm extended.

form 2.2

The transfer of weight between one leg and another is one of the key moves in t'ai chi. As the weight shifts onto one leg, it is said to be full. When a leg is not carrying weight, it is said to be empty. Although it is tempting to lean, remember to keep the body upright throughout the turning movement.

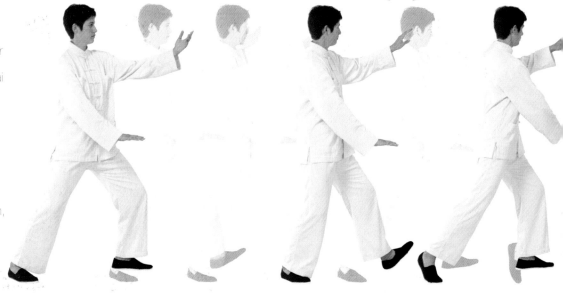

● Sit back on to your right foot, lifting the left toes and turning the body towards 7.30. As you do so, start to turn the left palm downwards.

● Transfer your body weight forwards onto your bent left leg, moving your foot towards 7.30. Move your right arm over to the left so that the hand is over the bent left knee, and start to turn the right palm upwards.

● Draw your right foot in as you finish turning the right palm upwards so you are holding the ball again.

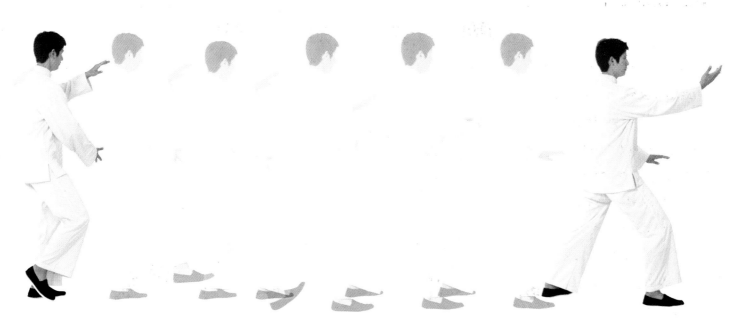

⬤ Step out with the right foot as though on railway lines, and place your right heel at nine o'clock. Your left leg should remain bent at the knee.

⬤ Transfer your weight onto your right leg, bending your right knee and stretching your left leg, but not so that it is locked.

⬤ As you move forwards, change the position of your hands. Extend your right hand so the palm is facing diagonally upwards.

⬤ Push your left hand down so that the tips of the fingers are in line with the right knee (this mirrors the first Parting the Wild Horse's Mane).

▶   ▶   ▶   turn to 9 o'clock   ▶

form 2.3

This form involves a change between the Left and Right Bow stances. You can practise this important transition on its own (see Introduction). Throughout this exercise it is important to control your movements and remain balanced so that you do not 'fall' into a posture.

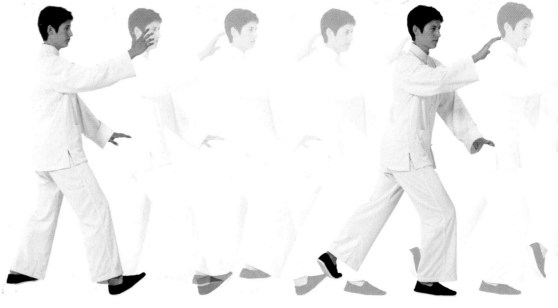

● Sit back on to your left foot, lifting the right toes and turning the body towards 10.30. As you do so, start to turn the right palm downwards.

● Now transfer your body weight onto your bent right leg, which points at 10.30. Move your left arm over to the right so that the hand is over the bent right knee, and start to turn the left palm upwards.

● Draw your left foot in as you finish turning the left palm upwards so you are holding the ball again. Step out with the left foot, as though on railway tracks, and place your left heel at nine o'clock. Your right leg should remain bent at the knee.

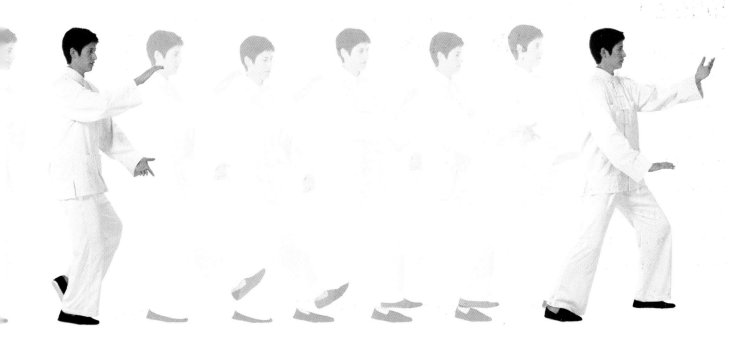

● Transfer your weight onto your left leg as you place your left toes on the floor, bending your left knee and stretching your right leg, but not so that it is locked.

● As you move forwards, change the position of your hands. Raise your left hand so the palm is facing diagonally upwards.

● Push your right hand down so the tips of the fingers are in line with your left knee.

● Your left arm should be extended but soft at the elbow, with the palm facing up at 45 degrees. The right palm should be facing towards the floor.

form 3 stork spreads its wings

This is a small and controlled movement. In this form the body makes three turns. It is the turn of the body that controls the movement of the arms. In the final posture, make sure your arms assume arc movements; as you raise the right wrist, concentrate on sinking the right shoulder and bowing both arms.

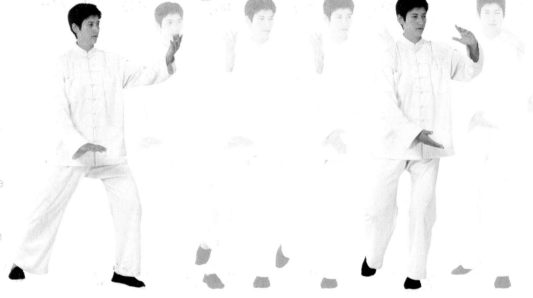

● Start from the position of parting the wild horse's mane at nine o'clock. Your left hand should be raised up with the palm facing in towards you, and your right hand should be lowered with the tips of the fingers in line with the left knee.

● Turn your body towards 7.30, and pick up your right foot and take half a step in towards your left foot. Put the ball of your right foot down, but keep the heel off the floor. Most of your weight should be on your left leg and your gaze straight ahead.

● As you step in, change the posture of your hands so you are holding the ball. The palm of your right hand should be facing to the sky and your left palm facing the ground. Your body should face 7.30.

face 9 o'clock ▶   **turn to 7.30** ▶

● Sit back onto your right foot and turn the body to the right as you lower the right heel so the foot points towards 10.30. Sit back onto the right leg and lower your left hand as you raise your right hand up.

● Your hands should meet at approximately heart height, with your left fingertips pointing upwards and brushing your right wrist crease. Your right fingertips should be facing to your left.

● Lower the left hand, with your palm down and your left fingers in line with the front of the left knee. Raise your right hand out to the side, level with the top of your head. It should be pointing diagonally upwards.

● Simultaneously, pick up your left foot, move it into your centre line with only the toes touching the ground. Continue to face forwards. The shoulders should be completely relaxed in the final posture.

turn to 10.30 ▶ **face 9 o'clock** ▶ **9 o'clock**

form 4.1

The final posture of this form is repeated three times: twice with the right hand extended, and once with the left. This form requires large circular movements with the arms. Remember that the outside arm should be well extended, but the elbow should never be hyper-extended or locked.

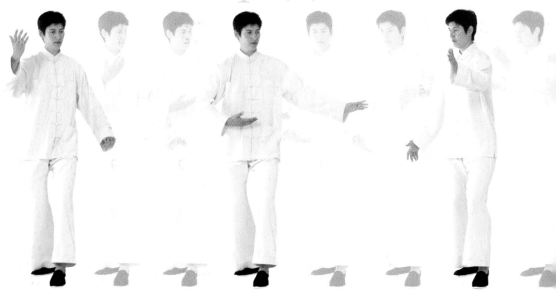

● Turn your body to the left as you move your right hand towards nine o'clock, turning the palm upwards. Having reached nine o'clock, begin to lower the back of the hand.

● As you lower your right hand, raise your left hand upwards. Your left fingers should rise to point upwards with the palm passing across the body at the height of your throat.

● Turn to the right as your right arm continues in a circular motion down and then up out towards 12 o'clock. Fold your left arm in so that the fingers are pointing at the elbow crease of the right arm, and your left thumb is opposite your sternum.

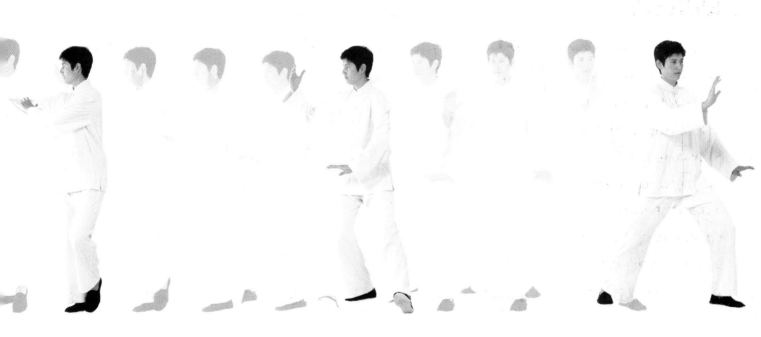

● Draw your left foot towards your right foot as you complete the previous arm movements.

● Fold the right hand in so that your right hand is level with your right ear. Simultaneously, push your left hand down the centre line of your body, and step your left heel out towards nine o'clock.

● Transfer your weight so that 70 per cent of it is on the left foot. At the same time, push your right hand out in front of you to nine o'clock. Sweep your left hand across from the centre line to the left side of your left knee with the palm down.

● The fingers are as far forwards as your left knee. Your right index finger is at the height of the tip of your nose, but slightly to the right.

heel to 9 o'clock ▶   face 9 o'clock ▶   9 o'clock ▶

Balance is important in this form – be aware of your weight distribution so as to avoid falling into a posture. When folding the wrist in towards the face prior to pushing, always keep the fingers and palm relaxed, and avoid lifting the fingers too high.

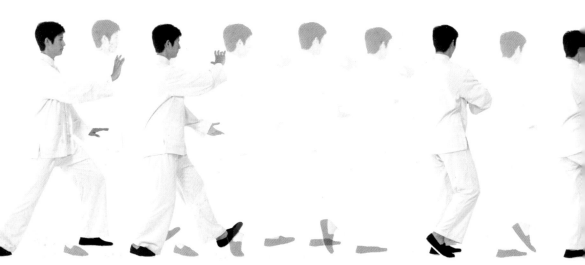

● Transfer your weight by sitting back on your right leg, as you turn your body to 7.30. Raise your left toe. Start to turn your left palm upwards.

● Move your weight on to your left foot, which is pointing towards 7.30. As your do so, bring the right foot into a T step movement. At the same time, raise the left arm out to the side; bend the right elbow so that the right fingertips point at the left elbow.

● Fold the left hand in so that it is level with your left ear. Simultaneously, push your right hand down the centre line of your body, and step your right heel out towards nine o'clock.

turn to 7.30

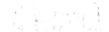

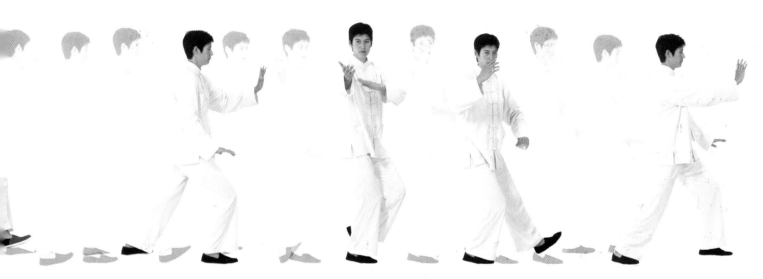

● Transfer your weight so that 70 per cent of it is on the right foot. At the same time, push your left hand out in front of you to nine o'clock. The fingers are as far forwards as your right knee. Your left index finger is at the height of the tip of your nose.

● Now sit back, lifting your right toes and turning to your right. Begin to turn the right palm up. Move your weight onto your right foot, drawing the left foot into a T-Step. Simultaneously, open the right arm out to the side with the palm facing up.

● Your left hand should be opposite your sternum with the palm facing downwards. Fold the right hand in towards your face, and push the left hand down your centre line. Place the left heel towards nine o'clock.

● Now push your right palm to nine o'clock as you transfer your body weight; the left palm should move out to the side and face down on the outside of your left knee.

heel to 9 o'clock ▶ **face 9 o'clock** ▶ **9 o'clock**

form 5 *playing the lute*

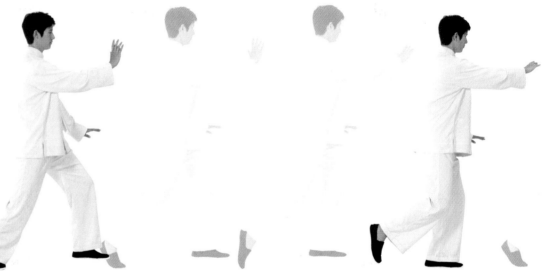

This movement involves a narrow stance in which most of the weight goes into the back leg, with the toes of the front foot carrying barely any weight. One of the applications of this move is to trap your opponents arms, with your left hand on their elbow, and the right on their wrist. Therefore, the distance between your palms is important.

● Turn your body to eight o'clock and move the right foot in half a step towards the left foot.

● Keeping your right arm extended and your left palm pointing towards the floor, allow the arms to move to the left with the turn of the body.

● Now sit back onto the right foot and turn the body to 10.30. Raise the left palm with the palm still facing downwards, and with the fingers pointing to nine o'clock.

turn to 8 o'clock ▶ ▶ ▶

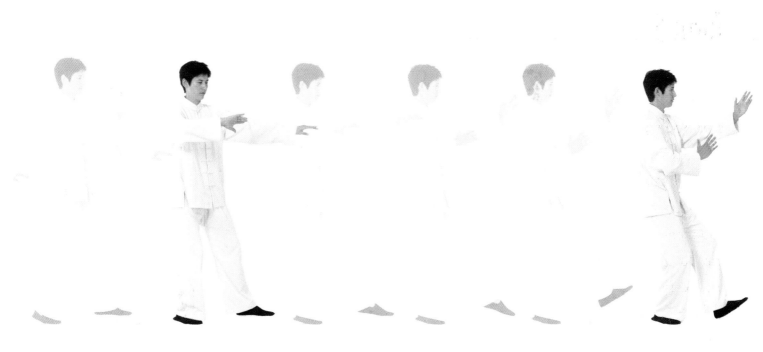

● Draw the right hand back, so that the back of the hand is opposite to your sternum.

● At the same time, rotate the right thumb downwards so that the palm turns away from the body. The middle finger and forearm should be in a straight line.

● Turn the body back slightly towards nine o'clock, and as you do so, rotate both thumbs upwards, so that the palm faces inwards.

● Simultaneously bring the left heel into the centre line to point to nine o'clock, with the toes raised. The right palm should face your left elbow crease, and the right fingers should point at your left wrist crease.

turn to 10.30   ▶   turn to 9 o'clock

form 6.1

repulse monkey (1 & 3)

Balance is extremely important in these four postures. When placing the foot behind you each time, don't put any weight onto the foot until you begin the 'push and pull' movement of the arms. During the 'push and pull', the upper hand passes over the top of the lower hand, but without touching it.

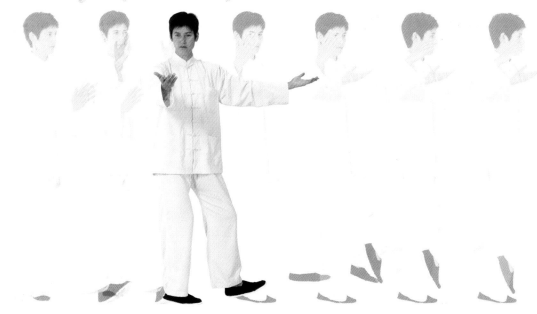

● From the Playing the Lute position, turn your body to the right so that you are facing 10.30. The right hand lowers to your pelvis and then rises to twelve or one o'clock.

● Extend the hand so that it is level with your left hand. Turn both hands so the palms are facing upwards.

● Fold the right hand towards the ear. Bring the left foot in towards the right, then step back, placing the toe directly behind the right foot, along your centre line. Your weight should still be on the right foot.

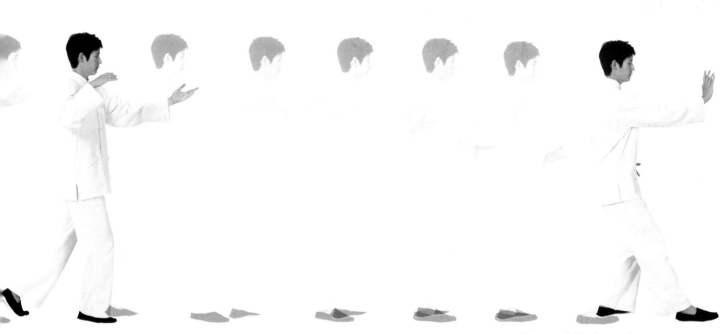

● Transfer your weight fully back onto the left foot and gently push forwards with your right palm as you slowly pull the left hand backwards to the left side of your pelvis. Your right hand should pass over the left without making any contact.

● As your weight fully transfers, adjust the front (right) foot, by allowing the right heel to rotate outwards.

● In the final position, the outer side of your left palm should rest lightly against the pelvic bone (towards the front of the pelvis). Your right hand should be pushing the palm away along the centre line of the body to nine o'clock.

● The feet are in an empty step. Check your stance as you come to this point in the form. The fingertips of your right hand should be in line with your nose.

▶ **face 9 o'clock** ▶

form 6.2

All four of these movements require the body to be turned to the left and right. Even whilst you are stepping the foot behind you, keep the body turned and only turn back to nine o'clock as you complete the 'push and pull' of the movement.

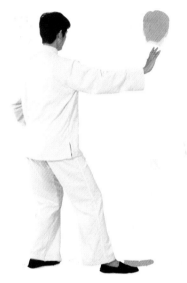

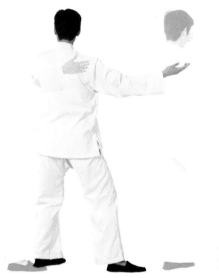

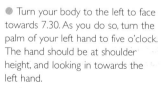

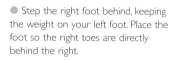

● Turn your body to the left to face towards 7.30. As you do so, turn the palm of your left hand to five o'clock. The hand should be at shoulder height, and looking in towards the left hand.

● Now fold the left hand towards the left ear as you bring the right foot in towards the left foot.

● Step the right foot behind, keeping the weight on your left foot. Place the foot so the right toes are directly behind the right.

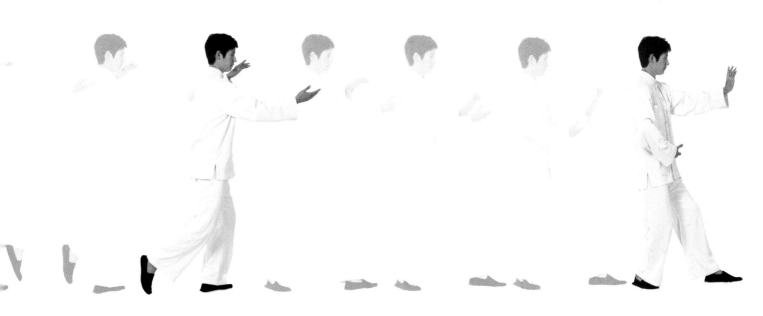

● Continue to hold your hands outstretched, with the palms facing upwards but soft at the elbows.

● Sit back onto the right foot. Push forwards with your left hand as you pull back on the right one. The left should cross above the right hand but without touching.

● Once your right hand has passed back under your left, bring it by the right hip, with the palm facing upwards. Leave a space between the side of your body and the elbow.

● Check that the tips of your fingers are in line with your nose. Now do Repulse Monkey again on both sides (that is, form 6.1 and 6.2).

form 7.1 *grasp the sparrow's tail (left)*

In the starting posture, make sure that your knee remains immediately above the 'substantial' foot – the one carrying the weight – and is aligned with your toes. In this posture, as in the previous four postures, it is very easy to allow the back knee to collapse inwards.

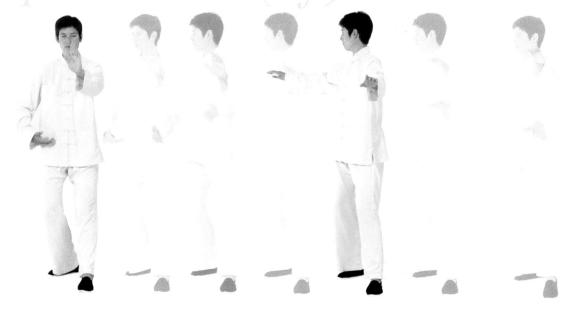

● Starting from the last posture in Repulse Monkey, turn your right hand palm face down with fingers in line with left knee. Turn your left palm inwards, with fingers at two o'clock.

● Rotating from the pelvis, turn your body to the right as you raise your right hand to face towards one o'clock. Both palms should be facing down towards the floor.

● Your body should be facing 11 o'clock, with the right foot facing out towards nine o'clock.

▶ hand to 1 o'clock   ▶ face 11 o'clock   ▶

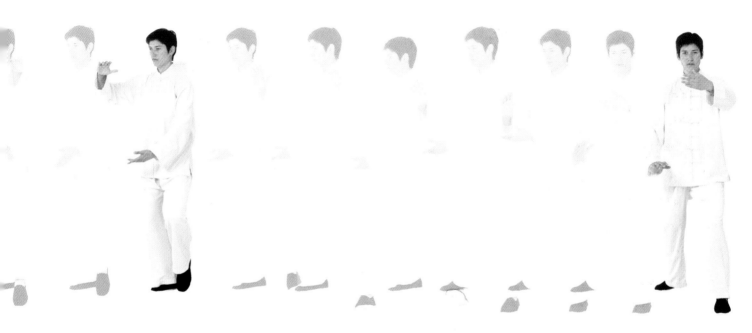

● Turn your body back slightly towards the left so you are facing 10.30. Let your right arm follow the movement of your body, and lower your left hand to fold it under the right hand.

● Fold your hands so you are holding the ball in front of the centre line, at the same time, bring the left foot into a T step.

● As you turn your body towards nine o'clock and transfer your weight to your left foot, raise your left hand with the palm facing in towards you, and push your right palm downwards.

● Your left hand should complete the movement at mouth height with the palm facing in towards your face.

turn to 10.30 ▶ turn to 9 o'clock ▶

form 7.2 *grasp the sparrow's tail (left)*

The waist controls the movement of the arms, so when the arms are moved to eight o'clock, it is the turn of the waist that makes it happen; they don't move by themselves. Make sure that the weight stays on the front foot immediately following Peng (or Ward Off).

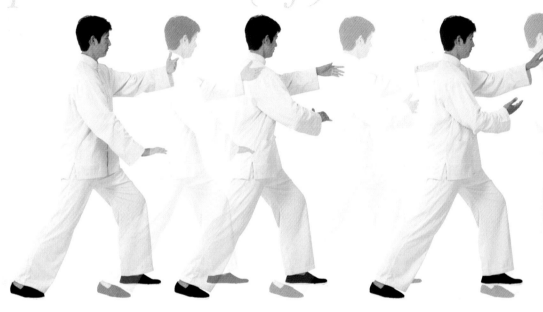

● This is called the Peng or Ward Off position. From this posture, turn the body slightly to the left, towards eight o'clock.

● Allow your arms to follow the movement of your body, and lift up your right hand with the palm continuing to face downwards.

● With the body still turned to eight o'clock, turn your left hand so that the palm is facing towards the ground. Turn your right hand so that the palm is facing up to the sky.

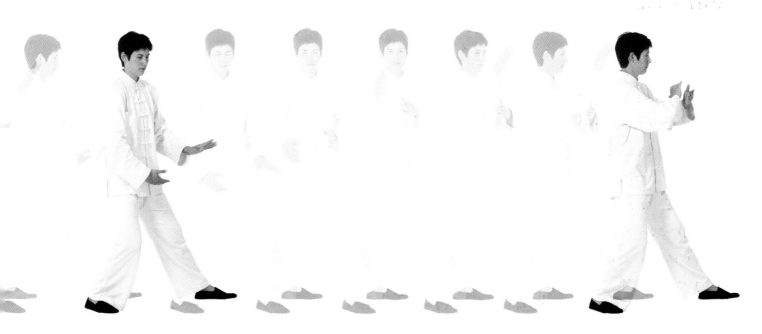

● As you transfer your weight back onto your right leg, slowly pull your hands down towards your body. This is called the Lu or Roll Back position. As the hands move towards the waist, turn to your right so that you are facing 10.30.

● Sweep your right hand out towards twelve or one o'clock, turning the palm to face nine o'clock. Simultaneously, turn your left hand to face your body and raise the hand up your centre line.

● Turn your body to face square to nine o'clock. At the same time, raise your right hand up to arc over and in front of your chest, folding at the elbow, with the palm continuously facing towards nine o'clock.

● As your right hand drops in front of your chest, it will meet your rising left hand, and the heels of both palms will connect. The weight is on the right foot throughout this part of the movement.

turn to 10.30 ▶ turn to 9 o'clock ▶

form 7.3 *the sparrow's tail (left)*

Keep the body upright throughout this sequence; to do this, make sure that there is a conscious transfer of weight from front to back to front foot. The pelvis should stay level throughout the movement. When sitting back, feel as though you are sitting into your rear heel.

● This move is called Ji, or Press. Transfer your weight forward as you press your arms out, with the heels of the palms still connected.

● Your arms are now outstretched and your body weight is 70 per cent on the front leg and 30 per cent on the back leg.

● Turn the palms downwards, and then 'wipe' the back of the left hand with your right palm. Separate your hands to a shoulder width apart and, sinking back onto your right foot, raise the left toes.

face 9 o'clock   ▶   **face 9 o'clock**

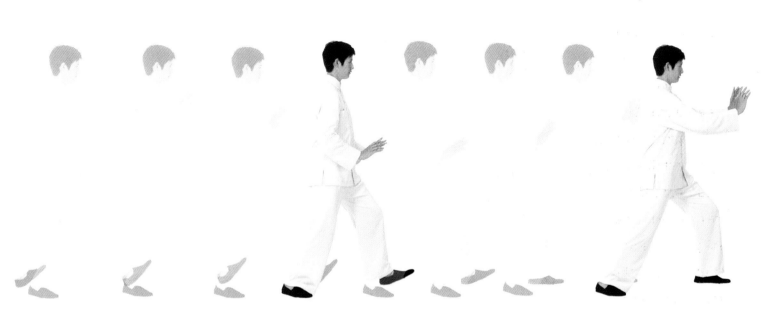

● Draw your hands back towards the chest, then push them down to your waist. Leave the fingertips slightly raised throughout the movement.

● Now move your weight forwards again and onto the left leg, bringing the left foot flat on to the floor.

● Lift and push the hands away from you to shoulder height, extending the arms but keeping them soft at the elbows.

● This final move in the form is called An, or Push Downwards (although the movement finishes by pushing ahead towards nine o'clock).

form 8.1 grasp the sparrow's tail (right)

As you turn to begin Form 8, keep your hands level. The left hand, although slower, should move from the left side to the right side at a constant rate; it should be in place as the upper hand in the 'hold the ball' position at the same time as the right hand arrives underneath it, and the right foot draws in.

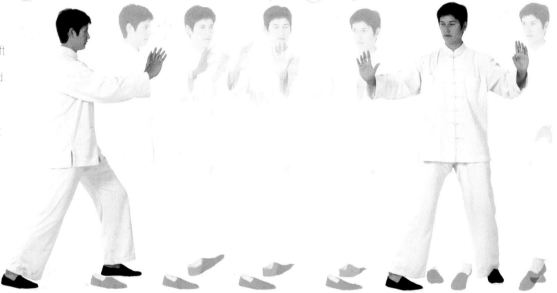

● Start this posture from the An or Push position. Your back should be straight and your gaze directly ahead. Move your weight back into your right foot, while at the same time lifting your left toes and turning your pelvis to the right.

● Turn the body towards 12 o'clock, pivoting the left heel and then placing the left toes so that they face 12 o'clock. As you turn your body, the hands will move with you, but allow the left hand to move more slowly than the right hand.

● Simultaneously move the right hand out towards 1.30. Keep turning the body as you transfer your weight back onto the left foot and lower your right hand.

face 9 o'clock   ▶   **turn to 12 o'clock**   ▶

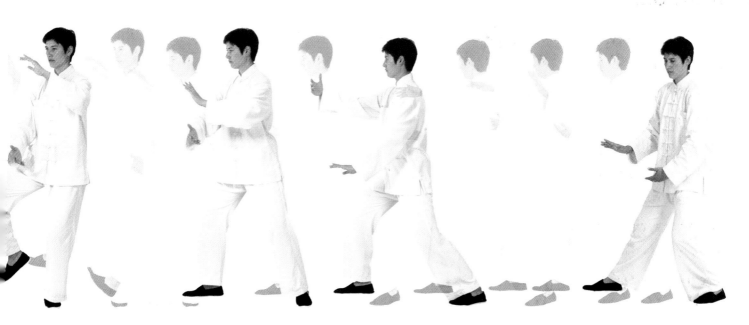

● Turn your body towards 1.30. Rotate the palm of your left hand down, and turn the right palm up, so that the hands are in the 'hold the ball' position. Draw your right foot back into a T-Step.

● As you turn your body towards three o'clock and transfer your weight to your right foot, raise your right hand with the palm facing your mouth and push your right palm downwards. Slip your rear heel as you complete the movement.

● From Peng, or Ward Off position, turn the body to the right, allowing your arms to follow the movement of your body. Now turn your right hand so that the palm is facing towards the ground and rotate your left hand so that the palm faces upwards.

● Now transfer your weight back onto your left leg and slowly pull your hands down towards your waist. This is called the Lu or Roll Back position. As the hands move towards the waist, turn slightly to your left so that you are facing towards 1.30.

turn to 1.30   **turn to 3 o'clock**   ▶   **face 1.30**

form 8.2 *the sparrow's tail (right)*

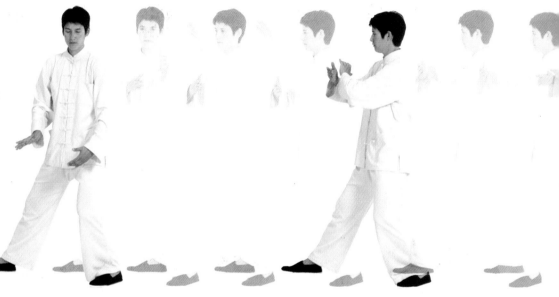

As you continue this movement, make sure your hips are level. When lowering the hands in the Lu position, it is very easy to inadvertently lean the body. Always be aware of the crown of your head and the vertical axis. When lowering your hands to your waist in Lu, maintain a space under both armpits, and avoid squeezing the arms into the sides of the body.

● Sweep your left hand out towards 11 or 12 o'clock, turning the palm to face three o'clock. Simultaneously, turn your right hand to face your body and raise the hand up your centre line.

● Now turn your body to face square to three o'clock. At the same time, raise your left hand up to arc over and in front of your chest, folding at the elbow, with the palm continuously facing away from the body.

● As your left hand drops in front of your chest, it will meet your rising right hand, and the heels of both palms will connect. Press your arms out and transfer your weight forwards, with the heels of the palms still connected. This move is called Ji, or press.

▶ turn to 3 o'clock ▶

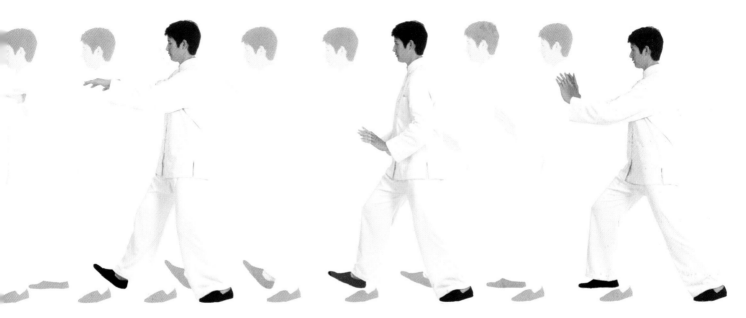

Your arms should be outstretched and your body weight onto your front leg. Turn the palms downwards and 'wipe' the back of the right hand with your left palm. Separate your hands to shoulder width, sink back onto your left foot, and raise your right toes.

Draw your hands back towards the chest and then push them down towards your waist. Leave the fingertips raised throughout. Now move your weight forwards again and onto the right leg, bringing the right foot flat on to the floor.

Lift and push the hands away from your body to shoulder height, extending the arms but keeping them soft at the elbows.

This final move in the form is called An, or Push Downwards (although the movement finishes by pushing ahead towards three o'clock).

face 3 o'clock

form 9.1 *single whip*

The twist of the body is important in this move, and it is essential that you don't allow the left foot to turn as you rotate your body to the left at the start of the form. Keep the upper hand relaxed as though brushing something away to your left side, and do the same with the right hand when it moves across to your right side.

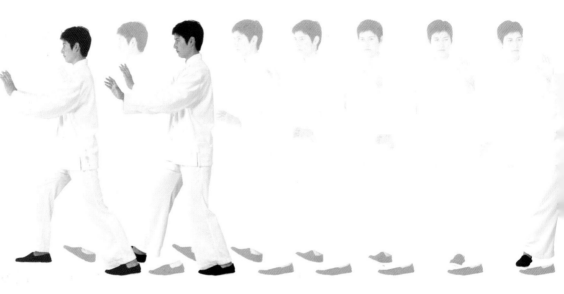

● Slowly transfer your weight back to your left leg, while still facing towards three o'clock.

● With your weight on your left foot, pivot your body to face 11 o'clock. Lift the toes of the right foot and turn them to 12 o'clock.

● Lower your right hand and push with the palm at pelvis height to 11 o'clock. Allow the left hand to move with the turn of the body to 11 o'clock.

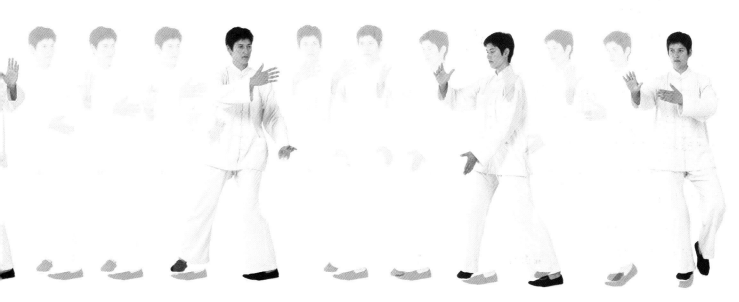

⬤ With your weight still on the left foot, change your hands over by lowering the left hand and raising the right hand up to throat height, with the palm of the right hand facing inwards. Your left foot should still be facing 1.30.

⬤ Now push your left palm towards one o'clock and allow the right hand to move to the left with the turn of the body. As you reach the left corner, the right hand turns with the palm facing away.

⬤ Now draw the left foot into the right in a T-Step. Lift the left palm up, bringing it towards the right wrist.

⬤ The fingers of your left hand should be pointing at the crease of your right wrist, with the left palm facing inwards towards the body. The right palm should face outwards.

turn to face 11 o'clock ▶ **turn to face 1 o'clock**

form 9.2

single whip

Keep the shoulders relaxed when moving into the Whip, particularly the right shoulder. Pull the Crane's Beak well in, thereby exposing the wrist. In certain applications, this can be used as a striking unit. Sink into your right foot, bending the right knee to make the turn.

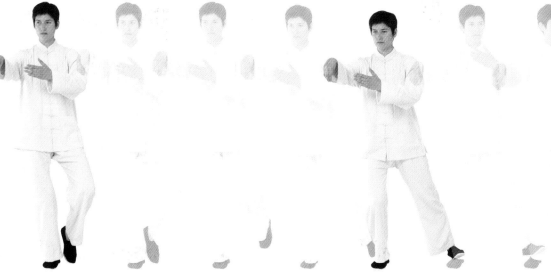

● Now push your right hand out towards the right corner. Bunch the tips of the fingers and thumb of your right hand together to form a single point.

● Flexing at the wrist, hook the fingers downwards to form the Crane's Beak posture. At the same time, step your left heel back diagonally towards eight o'clock.

● Now transfer the weight onto the left leg. As you do so, turn the toes to nine o'clock. As the weight transfers, 70 per cent will move to the left leg into a Bow Stance.

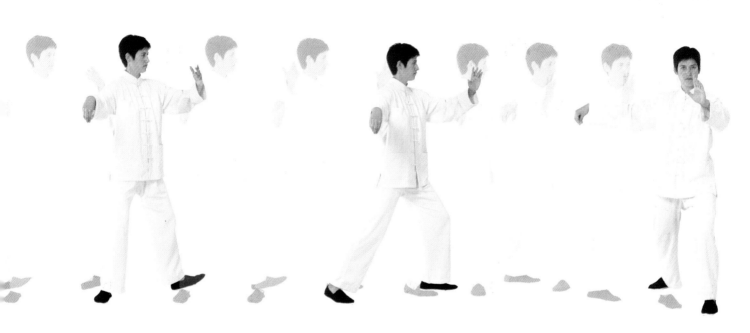

● At the same time, move the left hand from the left corner. During the left arm movement, the palm starts to turn away. Rotate the wrist to face the palm outwards towards nine o'clock.

● Throughout the movement, the right arm should remain extended with the hand formed in the Crane's Beak position.

● As you finish the movement, slip the heel of the right leg backwards, with the toes pointing approximately to 10.30.

● Push the left knee forwards with the toes pointing towards nine o'clock. The fingertips of the left hand should be raised so that they are in line with the tip of the nose.

form 10.1 *hands like clouds*

The arms appear to do a great deal of movement in this sequence, but in fact, relative to the body, they do very little. It is therefore important to turn the body to left and right – to the six 'corners'.

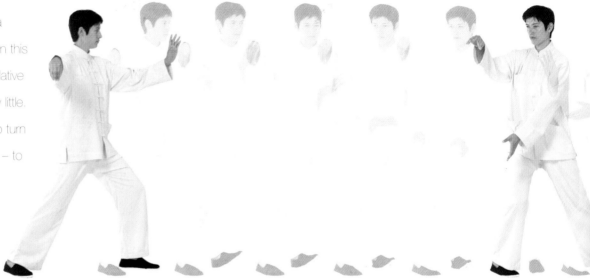

● From the Single Whip position, move your weight back onto your right leg and pick up your left toes.

● As you turn your body to the right, lower your left hand, pushing the palm down and across to the right corner. Pivot on your left heel, turning your left toes to 12 o'clock. Don't move the right toes.

● Once you arrive at the right diagonal, open up your right hand and turn your palm so it is facing away from you. Your left palm should be facing upright. Your weight is on the right foot.

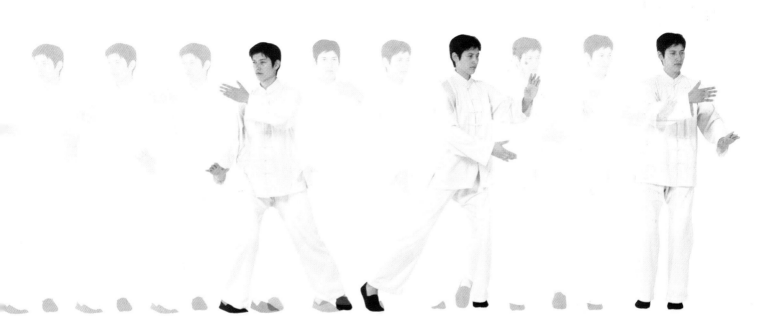

● With the weight still on your right foot, begin to change the position of your hands.

● Lower the right hand to hip height and raise the left hand so your palm is facing your throat.

● Take your weight onto your left leg as you turn your body towards the left. Simultaneously, push your right palm at hip height to the left corner. Then turn your left hand so the palm is facing away from you.

● Step your right foot in so that it lies parallel to the left, a fist width apart. Change your hands, lowering your left and raising your right.

face 1.30 ▶ **turn to 10.30** **face 12 o'clock** ▶

form 10.2 *hands like clouds*

For this part of the sequence, try to visualize the movements of the arms as two circles that move in opposite directions. Your right hand will move clockwise, while your left hand will move anticlockwise. Make the circles smooth and continuous, coordinating the stepping with the corners..

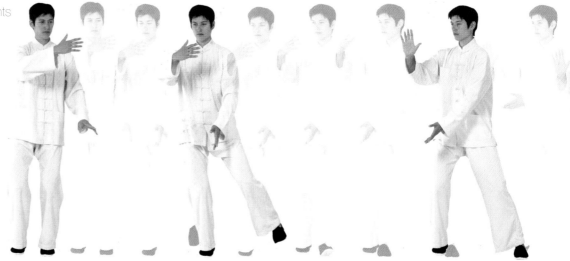

● Slowly take your body weight onto your right foot and turn to the right as you lift your left heel up.

● Step out with the left leg and begin to push your left palm across at hip height to the right corner.

● As your left hand reaches the right corner, turn your right palm away from you. It should remain at throat height. Your weight is still on your right foot.

▶ **turn to 1.30** ▶ ▶

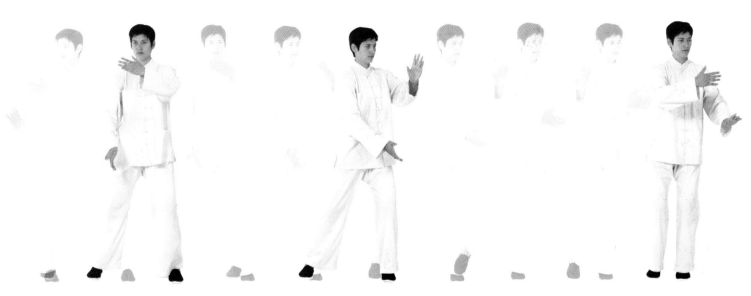

● Begin to change hands so that your left hand comes up on the inside of your body, palm facing towards you. Lower your right hand to hip height.

● Move your weight onto your left foot as you push your right palm at hip height across your body to the left corner.

● Once your right hand reaches the left corner, turn your left hand so the palm is facing away from you.

● As you turn your left palm away, begin to step your right foot in towards your left foot, a fist width apart.

form 10.3 *hands like clouds*

Keep your shoulders completely relaxed during this movement. It may be tempting to lift the shoulder of the rising hand, but try to allow the shoulder joint to relax. It often helps if you think of relaxing the shoulder *blade* rather than the top of the shoulder itself.

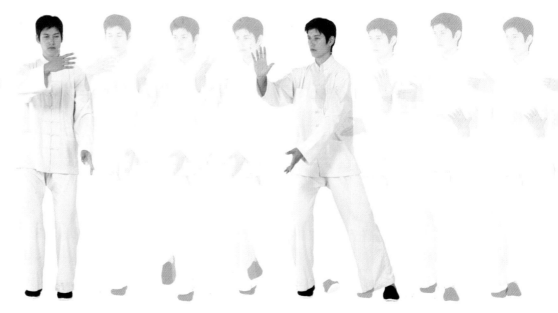

● As you move your weight onto the right leg, pick up your left foot and step it out shoulder width apart from your right.

● Push your left hand at hip height until it reaches the lower right corner. Turn your right hand so the palm is facing away from you at throat height.

● Keep most of your body weight on your right leg as you change hand positions. Lower your right hand and raise your left hand.

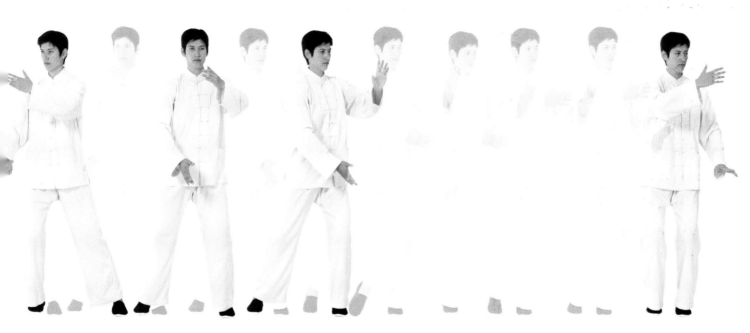

● Once your right hand is at hip height push your palm towards the left corner as you slowly transfer your weight to your left.

● Turn your left hand so that the palm is facing away from you and begin to change hands again.

● Bring the right foot in as you lower the left hand, palm facing downwards, and raise the right hand.

● Finish the Cloud Hands sequence with your left hand at hip height, palm facing down, and the right hand at throat height, palm facing you.

turn to 12 o'clock   turn to face 10.30   ▶   ▶

form 11

This is the second time that this movement appears. It is another form in which the shoulders are likely to rise; take particular care at the end of the form in the final posture – the right shoulder should be relaxed.

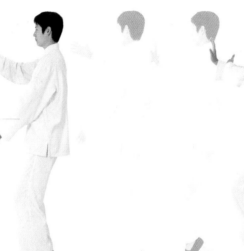
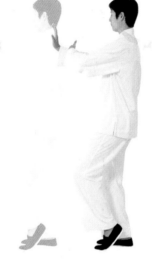

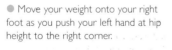
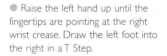

● Move your weight onto your right foot as you push your left hand at hip height to the right corner.

● Raise the left hand up until the fingertips are pointing at the right wrist crease. Draw the left foot into the right in a T Step.

● Push your right palm out, bunch the fingertips and thumb together and hook the wrist as before.

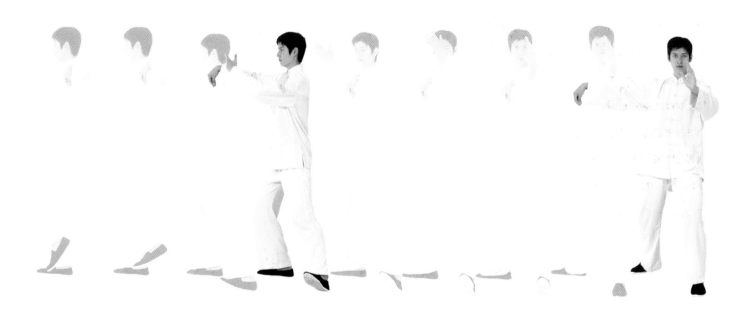

● The right hand therefore forms another Crane's Beak. The wrist should remain at shoulder height.

● Step your left foot backwards on the diagonal to eight o'clock, with the weight still on the right foot.

● As you transfer your weight to the left foot, make a sweeping arc motion with your left arm, while at the same time turning the left toe and your body towards nine o'clock.

● Turn your left palm away from you as you place your left toe. As you reach the end of the move, slip the rear heel. Your body weight should be 70 per cent forwards and 30 per cent backwards.

▶ **turn to face 9 o'clock** ▶

form 12 *high pat on horse*

The final hand posture in this move is similar to Repulse Monkey, but with one difference: the left palm doesn't draw back as far. One application of this posture is to control an opponent's right elbow with your left hand, whilst simultaneously striking at him with your right hand.

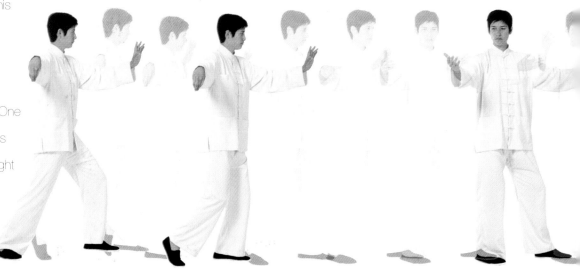

● From the Single Whip position, take half a step forwards with the right foot and turn your body to your left.

● Place the right toe down first, then place the right heel on a diagonal so that your foot is at a 45 degree angle away from your body. Your right foot will point towards 10.30.

● Turn both palms towards the sky as you sit back on the right leg and turn your body to the right. Look beyond your right hand.

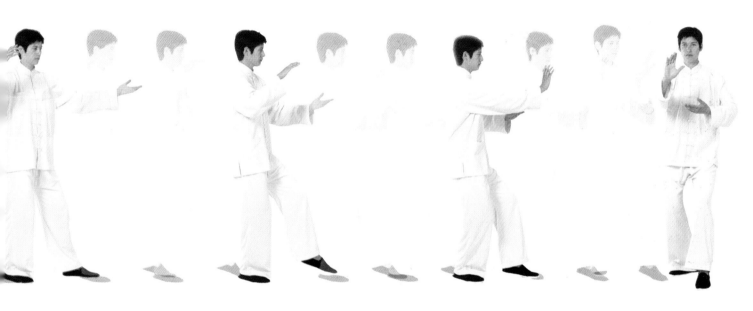

● Bend your right elbow so your right hand comes up by your ear. Keep your right hand relaxed and the palm facing diagonally downwards.

● Slowly push forwards with the right hand. At the same time, draw the left hand back towards you, with the palm facing the sky.

● As the push finishes, pick up the left foot and place the toe down ahead of the right heel. Keep the left heel off the ground.

● Push forwards with the right hand. The fingers of your left hand should be slightly below your right elbow. Keep your weight on your right foot.

face 9 o'clock ▶ **face 9 o'clock**

form 13.1

In the first part of this move (see the first three pictures), there should be a feeling of pushing down with your right hand, followed by the fingertips of the left hand leading towards a diagonal – as though slowly striking with them. But keep the hands very soft throughout.

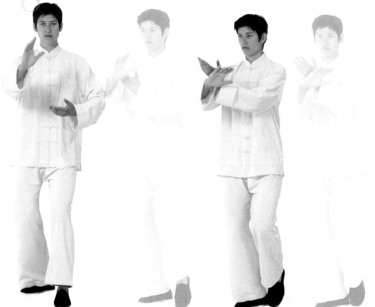

● From High Pat on Horse posture, slowly turn your body to the right and allow the right wrist to relax so that the palm is parallel to the floor.

● Slide your left hand up and over the right so that the backs of both hands are facing each other. The left fingers are at the height of your throat, with the left palm facing upwards. Draw the left foot into a T Step.

● Begin to turn your left hand so that the palm is facing away from you. Step the left foot out, placing the heel down first.

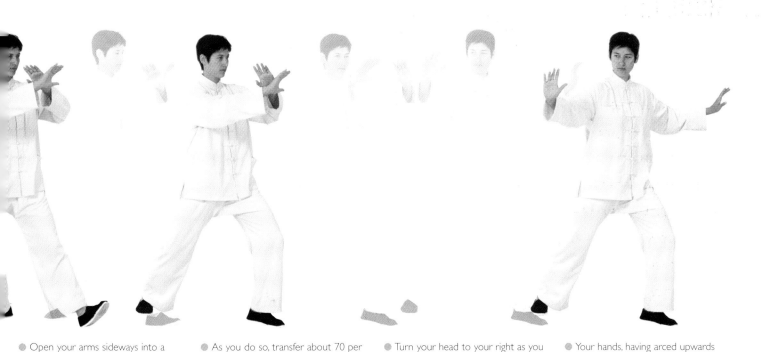

● Open your arms sideways into a wide arc. Turn your hands so your palms are facing away.

● As you do so, transfer about 70 per cent of your body weight onto the left leg and slip the right heel back.

● Turn your head to your right as you open your arms; your eyes should follow your right hand. Keep your fingers raised.

● Your hands, having arced upwards and opened, should lower to shoulder height, with the palms facing away from the body.

face 7.30 ▶

kick with right heel

When raising your leg, remember to relax your shoulders: this will help you maintain balance and allow your energy to sink into the standing foot. When crossing the hands in front of you, avoid leaning forwards; therefore you should feel the crown of the head 'suspending' you, with a direct vertical line to your front foot.

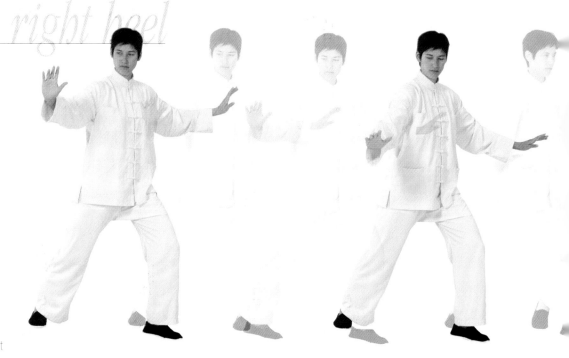

● Slowly lower your hands in front of your body. The weight will move increasingly onto the left foot.

● As the hands reach waist height, turn your head to face back in the direction of your right toes.

● Begin to lift your right heel off the floor and sink your weight forwards onto your left foot.

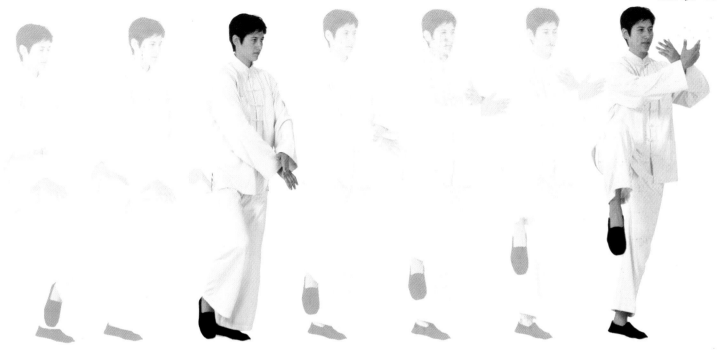

● Lift the right foot and keep your shoulders relaxed, while continuing to bring your hands together.

● Bring your right foot in towards the left foot, without touching. Cross your left hand over the right hand at the wrists in front of you.

● Raise your hands up towards your throat. Your right thumb moves under the left wrist so that your right hand is on the outside in the final position. Both palms should be facing inwards.

● As you raise your hands, also raise your right knee, as if it is being drawn up by the hands. Your right ankle should be relaxed. Keep the left leg straight, but not locked.

form 13.3

kick with right heel

This part of the form challenges your sense of balance, so you will need to relax your shoulders. Your left leg will be full, but you should mainly focus on your right leg and hand during the kick. Many beginners find the height of the kick difficult; try to kick as high as you can. If you have difficulty, kick to knee height first.

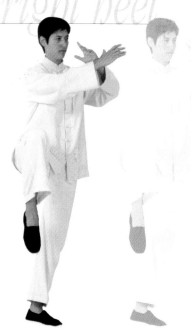

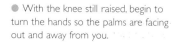

● With the knee still raised, begin to turn the hands so the palms are facing out and away from you.

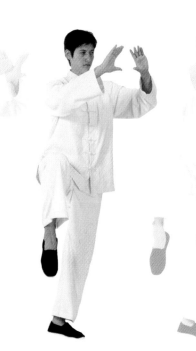

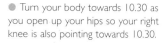

● As you turn and separate your hands, allow the palm of the left hand to wipe the back of the right hand.

● Turn your body towards 10.30 as you open up your hips so your right knee is also pointing towards 10.30.

● Maintain your balance on your left leg as your right toe continues to point towards the ground. Outstretch your arms, making sure the fingers are raised.

● Begin to straighten out your right leg as you kick the heel towards 10.30. Do not lean backwards when kicking, but keep your body upright.

● To keep your balance, concentrate on relaxing your shoulders and keeping your hips aligned.

● At the same time as the kick, extend your arms fully outwards. Make sure your right elbow is over your right knee and your left hand is pushing approximately towards 7.30.

body faces 9 o'clock ▶   **kick out to 10.30** ▶

form 14 *strike ears with fists*

When placing the right heel, it is important to bend your left knee to lower it rather than stretch the heel to the floor. In the final posture it may be tempting to raise the elbows, but think of this as a strike to the *underside* of the ears.

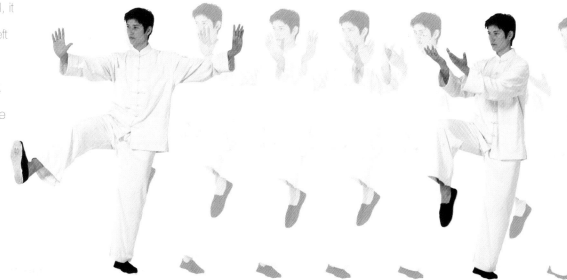

● Once you have kicked, bring your right foot back in towards your left leg. Keep your back straight and your shoulders relaxed, as this will help you maintain balance.

● Relax your right calf. Slowly bring your hands together until they are neck width apart. Twist the little finger edge of each hand towards you so that the palms are facing upwards.

● Keep your palms face up and bend your left knee. This has the effect of lowering your right foot to the ground.

● As you sink down, step out with your right heel. At the same time, lower your palms towards your waist. Keep your elbows out to the side of your body.

● As you start to transfer your body weight onto your right foot, separate your arms sideways in a circular motion, forming the hands into fists.

● Continue circling your arms up until they reach shoulder height. Relax your elbows and make sure that your palms are facing away from you, as they circle inwards to in front of your head.

● Slip your left heel backwards so your foot is at a 45 degree angle. The fists should be in line with your ears, with a head width between them.

right heel to 10.30   ▶   **body faces 10.30**   ▶   ▶

form 15.1

Ensure that your body stays upright as you make this turn, as it can be very tempting to lean. This problem can be minimised by keeping the arms level and the eyes (initially) on the left hand as it opens to seven o'clock; feeling that you are 'suspended' from the crown will also help.

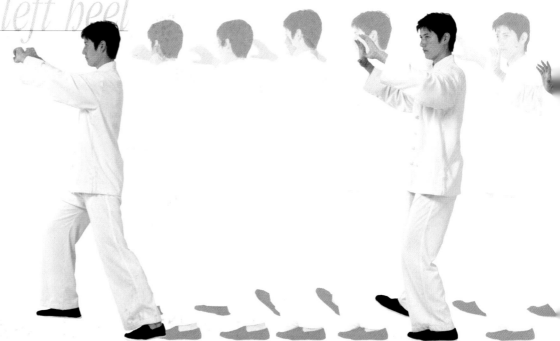

● From the Strike Ears with Fist position, begin to raise your right toe as you start to transfer your body weight backwards on to your left foot.

● As you move your weight onto your left foot, open your hands from the fist posture. Keep gazing between the two hands in front of you.

● Pivot on your right heel so that your body turns around to the left. Start to separate your hands.

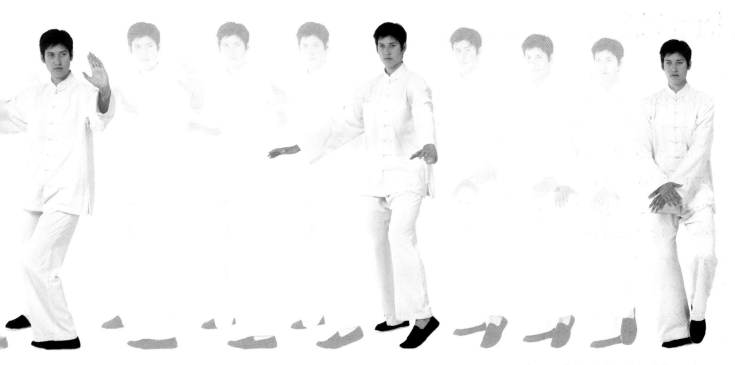

● Place your right toe down as far left as you can. Your eyes should follow your left hand around to seven o'clock. Your right palm should be facing away from you, approximately to nine o'clock.

● Sit back onto the right leg as you slowly lower your hands, with the palms starting to turn downwards and inwards to eventually face your body.

● Lift up your left heel and draw it in towards your right heel. Continue the downward movement with the hands, bringing them towards each other to cross at the wrists.

● Your left hand should be on the inside, closest to your body, and the hands should be crossed at the wrists.

form 15.2

In this form, keep the leg that you are standing on straight, but don't lock it at the knee. It will help your balance as you raise the left knee if you relax your shoulders completely and *feel* the foot on which you're standing. The eyes follow the main intention at the end of the move.

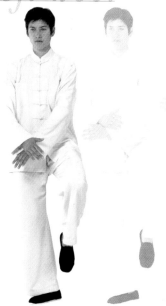

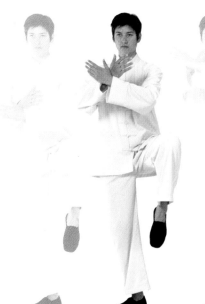

● Focus on keeping your balance as you transfer all your weight to the right leg and pick up your left heel. Relax your shoulders.

● Bend and raise your left knee to hip height. Make sure you keep the left toes relaxed. At the same time, raise your hands up your centre line.

● With your hands at throat height, gradually turn them so that the palms face away from you, still crossed at the wrists.

● Separate your hands, arcing them first up then outwards. Keep your fingers raised throughout this movement.

● Turn your hip out towards your left and let your eyes follow your left hand to your left side.

● As your arms arc out sideways and down to shoulder height, extend your right heel in a kick towards 4.30.

● Your eyes should now look beyond your left hand and the shoulders should be completely relaxed. Keep your right leg straight.

form 16.1

golden cockerel on left leg

The initial posture of this form is often known as Snake Creeps Down. This movement can be as physically demanding as you want to make it. Here, we show a medium height position, but you can sink much lower if you wish, or not so deep if it is too hard. This will depend entirely upon the strength and flexibility of your legs.

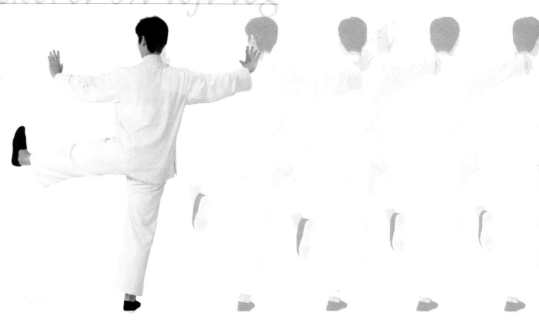

- Fully extend the left leg, keeping the toes pointing upwards. The left arm should be aligned with the left leg.

- Bend the right knee so your foot comes back in towards your right leg. Your knee should remain raised with your toes pointing to the ground.

- Keep your right wrist at shoulder height as you hook your right fingertips over to form the Crane's Beak.

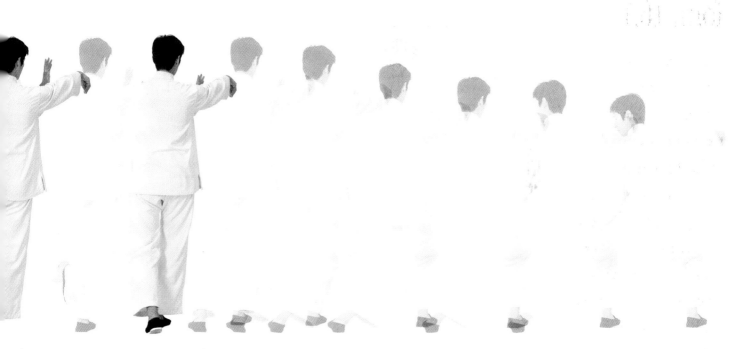

● Turn your body to the right as you arc your left arm over so that the palm faces your right elbow crease. Keep your left leg raised.

● Step back with your left foot so that you place the toes in line with the right heel. (This serves as a gauge to get the correct left foot/right foot alignment in the next move.)

● Maintain contact between the ball of your left foot and the floor as you slide your foot out to three o'clock. The toes of the left foot should remain in line with the right heel.

● Push the left palm down the centre line of the body. When it reaches waist height, thread the left fingertips to the inside of your left knee, with the palm facing towards six o'clock.

As you stand up onto your left foot into the Golden Cockerel posture, make sure that your left toes are turned outwards towards 1.30, as this will make it easier to balance on the single foot. In Golden Cockerel, feel the vertical line from the crown to the left foot.

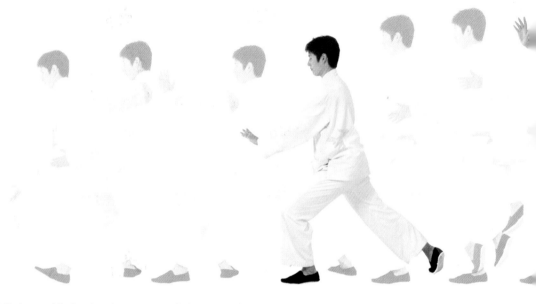

● Push your right foot into the ground as you move your weight forwards onto your left leg. Raise your left toes and turn them outwards towards 1.30. Simultaneously, start to raise your left hand ahead of you.

● As you transfer your weight to the left leg lift the toes of the right foot and turn them inwards. At the same time, drop the right arm down to your right thigh so that your Crane's Beak is pointing behind you.

● Raise your right knee so that you are standing on your left leg, and bring your right hand up in front of you. Your fingertips should be facing upwards and your palm to your left. Push down with your left palm.

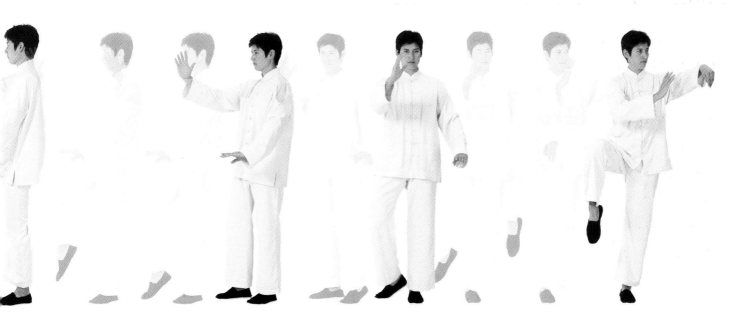

● Your left wrist should be flexed at hip height so that your palm is facing towards the floor.

● Lower the right foot so it is parallel to the left foot and also facing 1.30. Momentarily take your weight onto the right leg as you pick up your left heel and pivot it around so that the whole foot points to 12 o'clock.

● Move your weight back onto your left foot. Raise the left arm and form your hand into the Crane's Beak, as you raise your right knee.

● Arc your right arm across your body so that your right palm is facing your left elbow crease. Your eyes should look beyond the left wrist

form 17

Again, the initial movement is Snake Creeps Down. It is important to be very aware of your weight distribution. When sinking into the left foot at the start of this movement, keep the weight back as you slide the right foot out. This will ensure that you don't slide out too far.

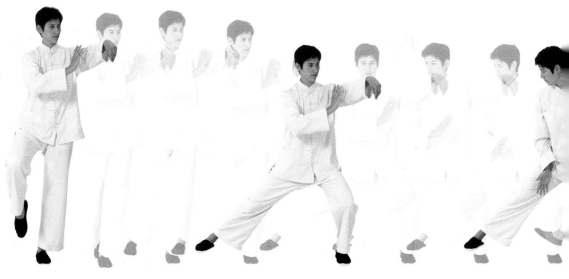

● Place the right foot behind your left foot so that the right toe is in line with the left heel.

● Slide your right leg out in a straight line to the right. Maintain your gaze out past the Crane's Beak of your left hand.

● Push your right hand down the centre line of your body to waist height, then thread the fingertips to the inside of your right knee.

face 10 o'clock ▶ **body faces 1.30** ▶

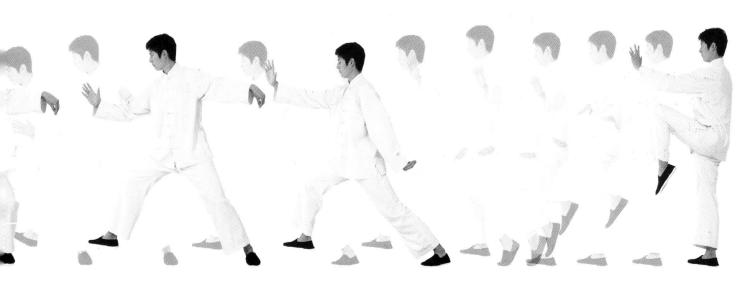

⬤ Turn the right toes out to 45 degrees. Take your body weight forward on to your right leg as you raise up your right arm so that your hand is at shoulder height.

⬤ Lift and turn the left toes so that they face towards 1.30. Turn your left hand as you lower the left arm to besides you, still in a Crane's Beak.

⬤ Your left wrist should now be facing the floor and the fingertips of your Crane's Beak pointing backwards. Shift your weight forward and your left heel lifts up off the floor.

⬤ Step onto the right leg as you raise your left leg so that your knee is higher than your waist. Draw your left arm up, palm facing outwards. Lower the right hand so the wrist is flexed and palm facing downwards.

form 18.1

As in Form 14, Strike Ears with Fists, when stepping forwards at the start of this form bend your right knee, rather than stretch the left heel forwards. The body rotates to the left diagonal and then 90 degrees to the right diagonal. Use the body to make the arm movements.

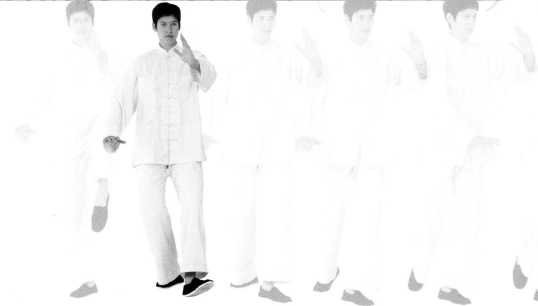

● Keep your hands in the same position as you bend the right knee – which will bring the left leg down – and then place the left heel in line with the right heel.

● Place the left toes down on a slight angle outwards. Begin to move your weight onto your left leg.

● As you do so, turn your body slightly towards the left. Begin to move your right hand under your left.

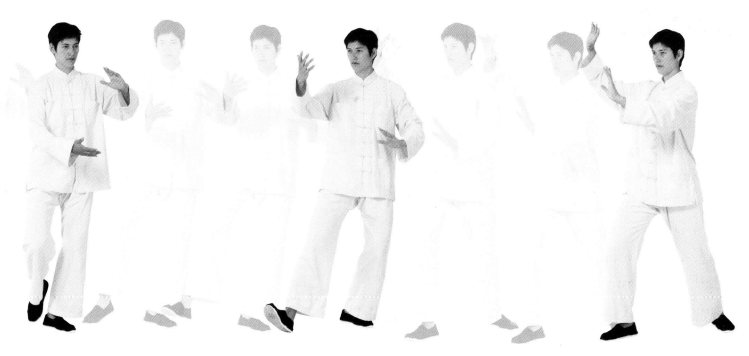

● Turn your right palm so you are Holding the Ball. At the same time, draw your right foot into your left.

● Step out to your left as you extend your right arm, sweeping the hand up and out towards 4.30. Keep all of your weight on the left leg.

● At the same time, bring your left hand down your centre line to underneath the ribcage.

● Transfer your weight onto your right leg. Turn the right palm away and move the hand upwards. At the same time, push the left hand away, palm facing away. As you complete the move, slip the rear heel.

▶ **turn to face 4.30** ▶ ▶

form 18.2

fair lady weaves the shuttle (left side)

This part of the form repeats the movements already completed on the other side. This creates a sense of balance within the form. Towards the end of the movement, as you extend the left arm with the palm up to the corner, initially keep the weight on the right foot.

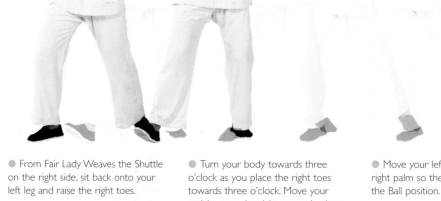

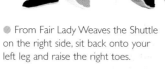

From Fair Lady Weaves the Shuttle on the right side, sit back onto your left leg and raise the right toes.

Turn your body towards three o'clock as you place the right toes towards three o'clock. Move your weight onto the right as you begin to lower the position of your hands.

Move your left palm under your right palm so they are in the Holding the Ball position.

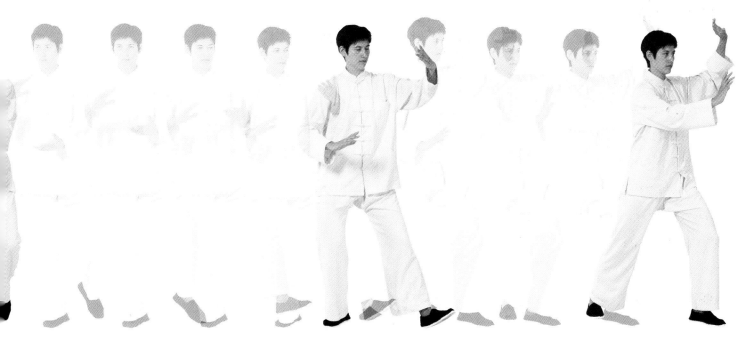

● Simultaneously, pick up your left foot and draw it into your right foot in a T Step. The foot should arrive as the 'ball' is formed.

● Keep your weight back as you place your left heel out towards 1.30. Extend your left hand out and up towards the corner.

● Turn and look towards this hand. As you do so, push your right hand down your centre line to below your ribcage.

● Transfer your weight onto the left leg as you turn both hands away. Move your left hand up and away as you push out with your right palm. Slip your right heel at the end of the movement.

form 19

There is less arm movement than there appears to be in this form; this is due to the rotation of the body from left diagonal, to right diagonal, to centre. Keep the neck in line with the spine to avoid letting the head drop.

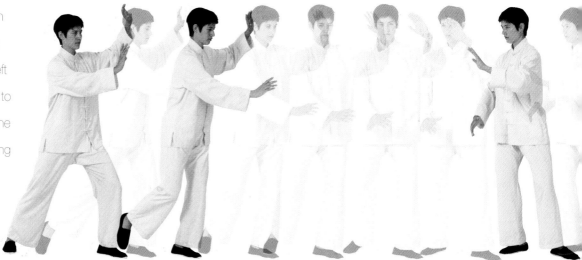

● From Fair Lady Weaves the Shuttle, pick up your right foot and bring it in towards your centre line. Start to move your weight onto your right foot.

● Begin to turn your body towards 4.30. Lower your right hand until it comes down to face your right thigh. Keep your right elbow and shoulder relaxed throughout the move. Your left hand blocks across your front to the 4.30 corner.

● Leading from the elbow in a circular motion, start to bring your right hand up towards your ear, whilst pushing your left hand down the centre line of your body.

face 1.30 ▶ **turn to 4.30** ▶

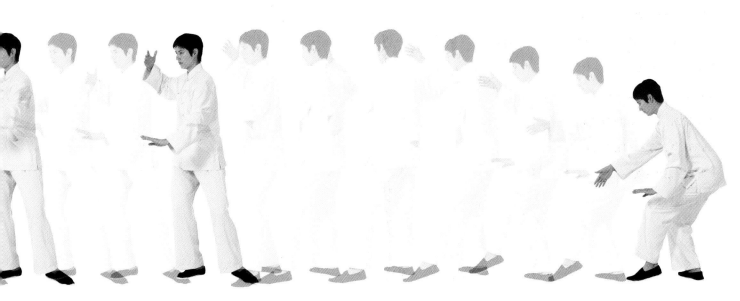

● Keep the right palm facing towards you as you take the hand up. The fingertips should be facing diagonally upwards.

● Your left hand should be flexed at the wrist, palm facing down. The weight is entirely on the right foot.

● Bring the left hand across, but above your left knee as you turn the body towards three o'clock. Your left toes should move into the centre line, towards three o'clock.

● Dive down with the right hand so that the little finger edge is pointing downwards at a 45 degree angle to the body. Keep your back straight and direct your gaze about a metre in front of your right hand.

turn to face 3 o'clock

form 20

Coordinate the raising of the hands with the movement of the body. You should feel as though it is your centre (Dantian) that is lifting your hands and pulling your foot inwards. As in Form 19, relax the shoulder of the raised arm.

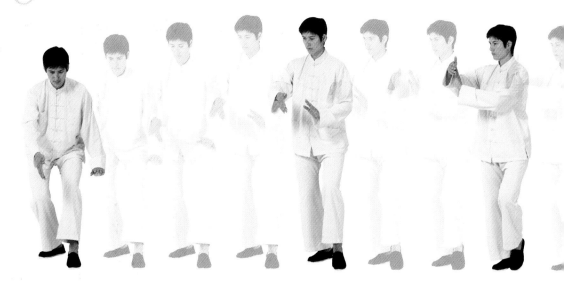

● From the three o'clock posture, stand up, with the weight still on your right foot and straighten your body.

● At the same time, raise both hands. Bring the fingers of the left hand to point towards the right wrist crease, approximately at chest height.

● Draw the left toes back to the centre in a T Step while maintaining the hand position.

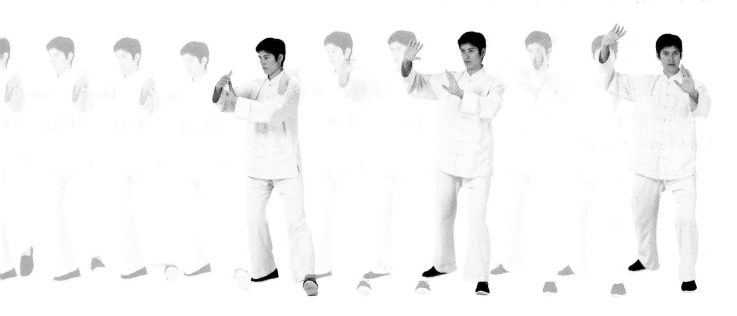

● Now place your left heel towards three o'clock, keeping your body weight on your right foot.

● Transfer your body weight onto your left foot. Now rotate your right wrist and turn your right palm out and away from the body, raising it up to head height as you do so.

● At the same time, push your left hand, with palm facing outwards, towards three o'clock. Raise your left hand until the tip of the index finger is level with the tip of your nose.

● Your right palm should be facing outwards towards four o'clock, while your left hand should be pushed forwards and further from the body. Your weight should be 70 per cent forwards in the Bow Stance.

▶   **turn to 3 o'clock**   ▶

form 21.1

In the first part of the form, make sure that the weight transfers completely onto the right foot. It is important to sit back onto your right foot first before turning your body past six o'clock. By doing this, all of your weight will be on the foot upon which you're rotating, and therefore you merely rotate on a vertical axis. Try to avoid leaning as you turn. Both hands should lift and arc as though tracing the outline of a rainbow, while the shoulders should remain relaxed. The finishing hand posture should mirror the starting hand posture.

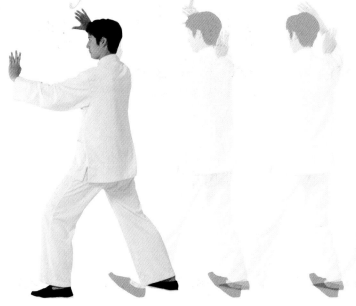

● Keeping your back straight and hips aligned, transfer your weight backwards on to your right foot.

● Now begin to turn your body towards 7.30, while at the same time lifting and turning the toes of the left foot towards six o'clock.

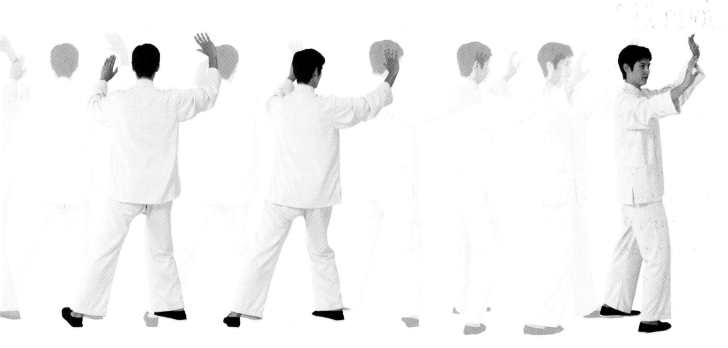

⚫ Simultaneously, in a broad sweeping movement, arc your arms over from the three o'clock position to 7.30.

⚫ Turn your body to the right to face 7.30 and place your left toes on the floor. Your body weight should remain on the right foot throughout this movement.

⚫ Continue the movement until your head is facing towards 7.30, with your eyes looking beyond your right hand.

⚫ You will notice that the final position of the hands mirrors the starting hand position.

turn to 7.30 ▶ **face 7.30** ▶

form 21.2

As with Form 14 (Strike Ears with Fists) and 19 (Needle at the Bottom of the Sea), bend your left knee in order to make the step ahead with the right foot. Don't try to stretch the foot out ahead of you. As you do so, tuck your tailbone under. An application of this move is to deflect a blow from an opponent while simultaneously striking back.

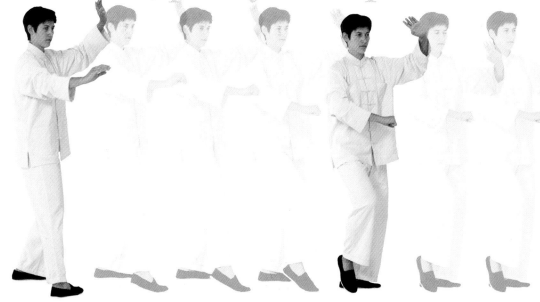

● Form the right hand into a fist with the palm of the hand facing downwards.

● As you form the fist, draw it downwards towards your waist. Keep the fist away from the body. Keep your left hand raised at head height with the palm facing away.

● Simultaneously, draw your right foot in towards the left foot in a T Step. Keep both legs bent at the knees.

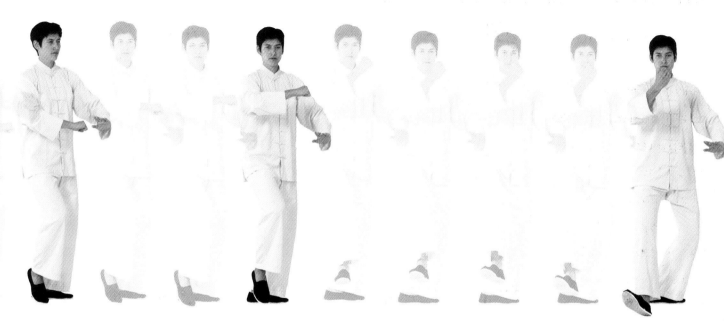

⚫ Then push your left palm down the centre line of your body to waist level. Almost immediately the right fist starts to rise.

⚫ To perform the deflecting movement, lift the right fist up to throat height, with the palm still facing downwards. As you do so, begin to lift your right foot.

⚫ Step your right heel out towards nine o'clock, turning the toes outwards. The back of the right fist should arc up the centre line and then down and away from you to point towards nine o'clock, with the palm of the fist facing in towards the body.

⚫ Your body weight should still be on your left foot. At the end of the move, your right forearm should be at a 45 degree angle, with the knuckles of the fist in line with your chin. The elbows should be relaxed and opened naturally out to the sides.

▶ **turn to 9 o'clock**   ▶

form 21.3 deflect downwards, parry and punch

This part of Form 21 contains the parry and the punch. After the deflection, the hands swing out to the sides, the body rotates and then the right hand punches as the body rotates back. Just as important as the hands are the movements of the feet and the shifts of weight. Be careful not to over extend the punch, as this will tend to push the shoulder forwards.

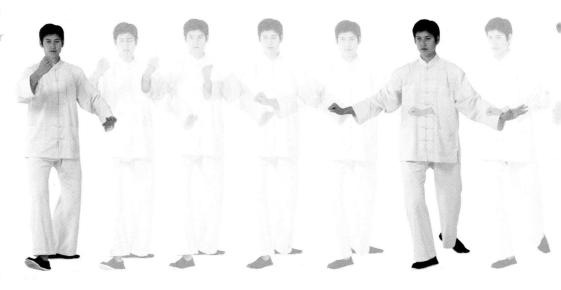

⬤ Lower your right toes onto the floor and take your weight forwards onto your right leg with the toes turned outwards.

⬤ As you do so, sweep your arms out to either side, keeping your right hand in a fist and your left hand open, palm facing the floor. Allow the elbows to drop and lower the hands below the level of the elbows.

⬤ Shift your body weight forwards as you bring your left foot into your right foot and turn your body around to the right. As you do so, your left palm should turn to face the right in a slapping motion.

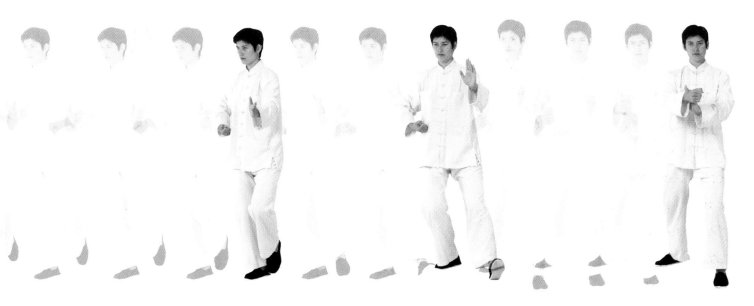

● Rotate your right fist with palm upwards to finish the move along the right side of the hip. At the same time, your body finishes turning to 10.30.

● Now move your left heel towards nine o'clock. Turn your left palm slightly away from the body, also to nine o'clock, and turn your eyes in the same direction.

● Now transfer your body weight forwards and onto your left foot, placing your left foot flat on the floor and into a Bow Stance. Punch the right fist forwards to nine o'clock, rotating the 'eye' of the fist upwards.

● The right elbow should be slightly bent. Draw the left palm backwards so that the palm faces the wrist of your right hand. Don't over extend the right arm.

turn to 10.30 ▶ turn to 9 o'clock ▶

form 22

Keep your whole body relaxed, in particular your shoulders and the palms of your hands. Note that your palms turn to face downwards as you draw them back towards your shoulders; the turn is often left until too late. Avoid leaning as you sit back onto the right foot and push the palms downwards.

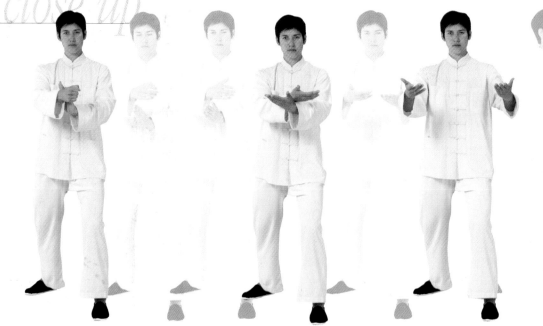

● With your body weight still forward on your left foot, trace the tips of the fingers of your left hand underneath your right wrist, turning the palms upwards.

● By the end of the move both palms should be turned upwards and crossed at the wrists, with the fingers pointing diagonally away.

● Now separate your hands so that they are a shoulder width apart, with the palms facing upwards.

face 9 o'clock   ▶   ▶

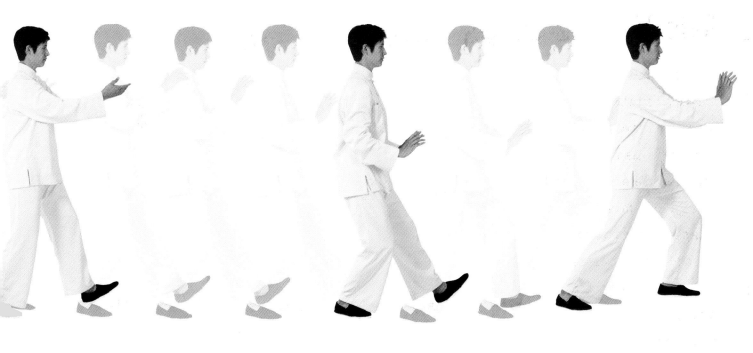

● Sit back and transfer your weight onto the right foot, lifting the left toe. Now draw the hands back towards your chest, turning the palms downwards when you are halfway.

● Continue by pushing the hands downwards as you complete the sitting back movement. By the end of the move the palms should have reached your waist. The wrists will be flexed back slightly.

● Slowly transfer your weight forwards as you begin to push your hands up and out. When pushing the hands out, they should be shaped as though pushing a large beach ball.

● Take your weight forwards onto your left foot as you gradually raise your hands to shoulder height. Your left knee should be in line with the tip of your toes. This is a Bow Stance.

face 9 o'clock ▶ **face 9 o'clock** ▶

form 23.1 *cross hands*

This move involves a double pivot of the feet – but not simultaneously; turn the left foot first, and then the right foot. The left hand makes less lateral movement than the right, and the coordination is important. Therefore the left hand needs to move slower than the right hand.

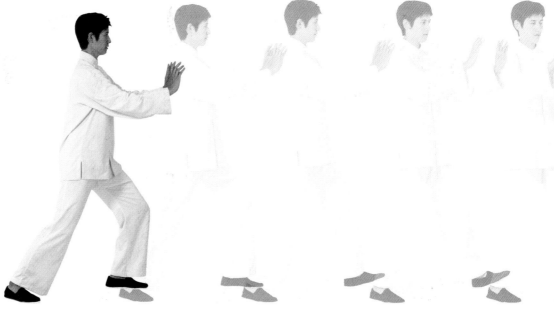

● Your weight should be distributed 70 per cent on the front leg and 30 per cent on the back leg, with your gaze straight ahead.

● Transfer your body weight so that you are sitting back on your right leg. Raise the left toe slightly.

● Keep your gaze in front of you as you turn your body towards the right and pivot right on your left heel.

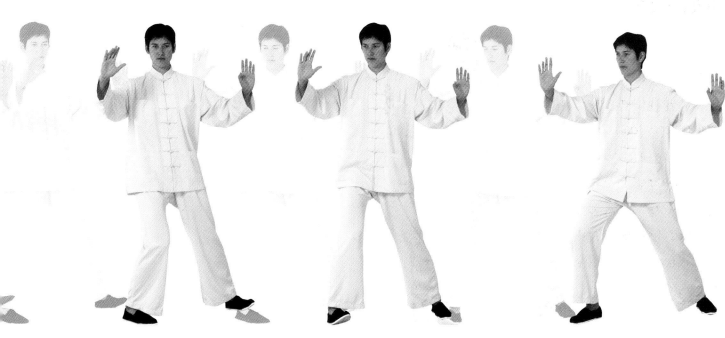

● As you place your left toes on the floor, pick up your right toes and move them towards 1.30 in a continuous transfer in body weight.

● Bring your right toes to rest flat on the floor, turning your head to the right to face 1.30.

● As you turn the body, the arms will move parallel to the ground with the left arm moving more slowly than the right arm, so that the gap between them gradually increases.

● Sink further into the right leg, making sure that your knee is in line with the foot and pointing to 1.30. At the end of the move, your right arm should face 1.30 and your left arm should face 11 o'clock.

form 23.2 *hands*

As you lower the hands, avoid any leaning – a common mistake. The right toes can be turned inwards towards 10.30 or only as far as 12 o'clock, but the reason for turning them inwards is that it avoids 'jumping' the right foot in when you draw it in to a shoulder width stance. Your ability to avoid this will depend on the strength of your left leg.

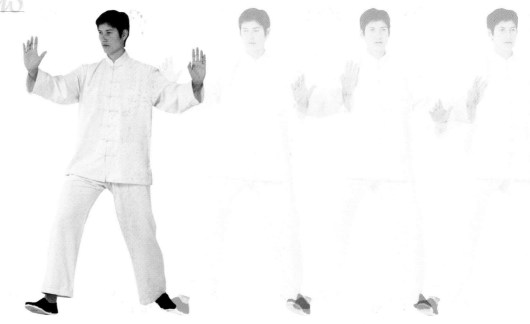

● Move your body weight back onto your left foot, lifting the toes of the right foot as you do so, and turning them inwards.

● Simultaneously start to lower your hands and turn your body to the left.

● Continue to lower your hands, sweeping them into the body so that at the end of the move the left palm crosses over the right hand. Both palms should be facing inwards.

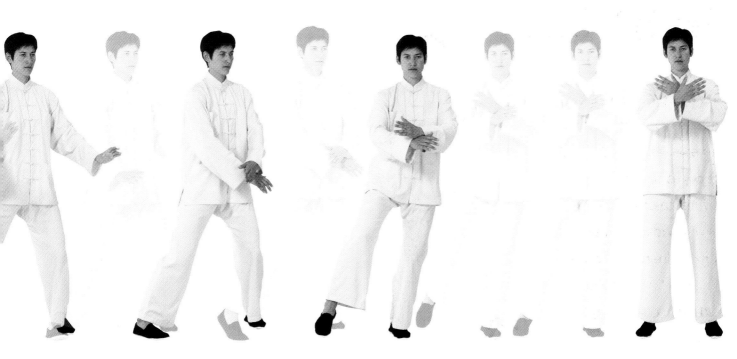

● With the weight still on the left foot, push onto your right toes and lift your right foot backwards to a shoulder width distance from your left foot. Avoid 'jumping' the foot inwards.

● As you do so, slowly raise your crossed hands and turn towards 12 o'clock.

● To raise your hands, move your right thumb under your left wrist so that, when raised, the right hand finishes on the outside, with both palms facing inwards towards the body.

● At the end of the move, you should be facing towards 12 o'clock, with your hands crossed at the wrists and facing the top of your chest.

turn to 10.30   ▶   **turn to 12 o'clock**   ▶

form 24.1

Keep the body completely relaxed, with the crown rising but shoulders sinking into your feet. Keep the wrists, fingers and palms soft and relaxed; also relax the back of the neck – with your hands in front, it is easy for the neck to become tensed. Breathe in a relaxed and comfortable way. As you start to lower the hands, allow the wrists to flex gently.

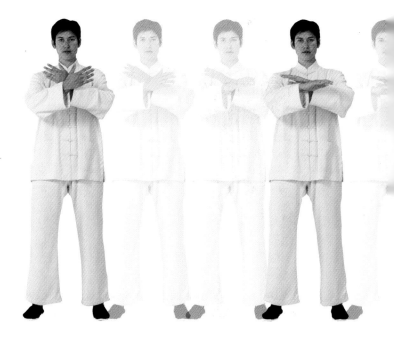

● Your feet should be a shoulder width apart, your back straight and your gaze straight ahead.

● Slowly turn your hands so that your palms are facing the floor. The left hand should be over the right and still connected at the wrists.

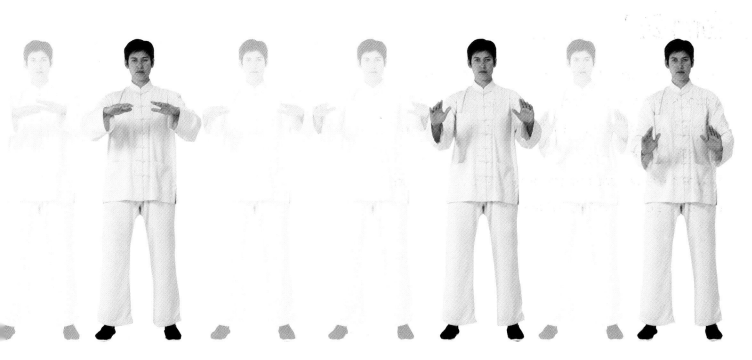

● Slowly separate your hands to shoulder width. At the same time, keep your shoulders level.

● Concentrate on keeping your spine straight, as if you were suspended by a thread from the ceiling. This will ensure that your neck is aligned too, but keep it relaxed.

● Once your hands are a shoulder width apart, lower your elbows and allow the hands to follow.

● As you do so, keep your wrists slightly flexed but relaxed and your fingertips initially pointing slightly upwards.

▶ **face 12 o'clock** ▶

form 24.2

closing form

This closing form is really a mirror of the stepping out procedure at the beginning of the form. When the hands have lowered, feel your weight in your feet. Be conscious of the weight transfer as you move your weight across to your right foot; fractionally before lifting your left toes off the floor, feel *all* the weight of the right foot, and the vertical line from the crown to the right foot, so that the entire spine feels connected.

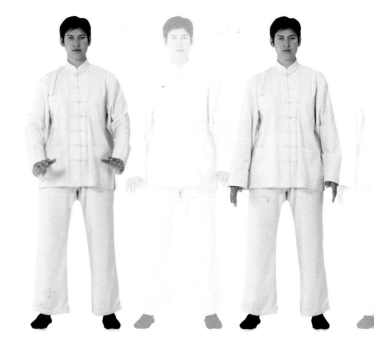

● Lower your hands towards your sides. Lower your fingertips until your palms face in towards your thighs, with the middle finger lined up with the seams of your trousers.

● Your fingers should be pointing towards the floor. Your body should be completely relaxed and soft.

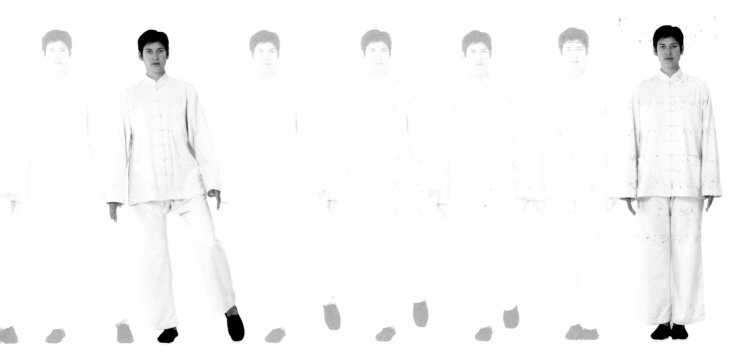

● Now transfer your weight onto your right foot. As you do so, allow the top of your head to rise so that you can feel a direct line running from the crown to the right foot. Feel your body stretching out and elongating.

● Pick up the left foot by first raising the left heel. Next, move the left foot in towards the right foot.

● Place the left toe down, followed by the heel. You should now be standing with your feet together.

● Continue breathing as you feel the connection from the top of the body down to your feet. You have now finished the form.

▶ **face 12 o'clock** ▶ ■

index

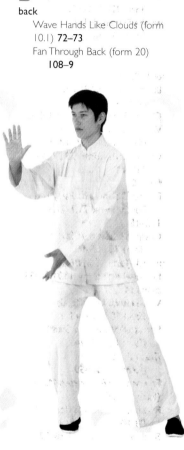

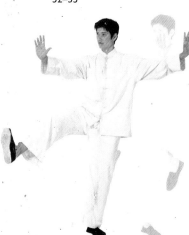